# Mainstay

## For the Well Spouse
## of the Chronically Ill

### MAGGIE STRONG

LITTLE, BROWN AND COMPANY   Boston · Toronto

FIRST EDITION

*Library of Congress Cataloging-in-Publication Data*

Strong, Maggie.
  Mainstay: for the well spouse of the
chronically ill.

  Bibliography: p.
  Includes index.
  1. Chronically ill — Home care.  2. Chronically ill —
Family relationships.  3. Adjustment (Psychology)
I. Title.
RA644.5.S77  1988      362.1′4      87-16873
ISBN 0-316-81923-9

RRD VA

*Published simultaneously in Canada
by Little, Brown & Company (Canada) Limited*

PRINTED IN THE UNITED STATES OF AMERICA

For Us

Because Francie said,
"Write a book for us. There's
a hundred books for them and not
a single book for us."

*

And for
Deborah
Seth
and
Ted
who know best

*

# Author's Note

The author wishes to thank the women and men who spoke forbidden words — may their publication give voice to others. I also thank the friends who encouraged me to do this book, and who kept me straight. Mostly, I thank my family for allowing themselves to be written about with the necessary combination of love and candor.

Many names and personalizing details, including location, have been changed to protect privacy. Only when a first and last name appear with a descriptive phrase or title may the reader take the name as an actual identification. Accordingly, if a doctor is referred to simply as "Dr. So-and-So," the true name is anything but that. And here I want to thank beneficent health professionals — some mentioned by full and some by partial names — for both their work and their contribution to this project.

Now for my agent, Molly Friedrich, who actually filled the Food envelope, and for my editor, Fredrica Friedman, who not only kept the whole book in mind unsullied but also flagged the early draft with more than one hundred absolutely valid yellow slips: bravo.

# Contents

(*Note:* Chapters with titles in italic type give Maggie Strong's personal account; chapters with titles in roman type present the stories of other spouses, practical suggestions, and analysis from various authorities.)

# Here's Who We Are

When I answer the phone, a woman's voice says, "How do you *do* it? I mean you've been doing it *six years*! I'm only a few months in and I'm going crazy, crazy!" It's Francie again, calling three thousand miles from Pasadena. On the day her older son flew east to start college, her husband was diagnosed with kidney failure.

Both journalists, Francie and I met years ago in Chicago while covering, ironically, a conference on stress. Podium talk about juggling the many hats of the working mother brought laughter and plenty of "Amens" from the audience. There was no mention of what I was going through, though — wearing all those hats, plus living with a chronically ill husband who needed to be assured about his manhood and his adulthood. I was alone and growing lonelier. I couldn't speak to my husband the whole of my sadness at what was happening to him or much of my sorrow at the loss of a life's companion, and nothing of my daily fear that I wouldn't be able to keep the kids in jeans or myself from eventually becoming like an older woman I knew who, when she turned her disabled husband over in bed, would sometimes "accidentally" scratch him with her fingernails.

"Seven years," I remind Francie. "And it was only this year I got my second wind. So tell me, what's happening?"

Some months my phone bill to the coast hits fifty dollars. It's worth it. What Francie is going through provides me with a backward glance at myself, lets me forgive myself for emotions that seem perfectly justified when they come from *her*, and shows me just how rocky our road is, and how far I've traveled. "God," Francie says. "Just knowing that you're intact is what's keeping me going."

"But I'm not intact," I tell her. "You never knew me before! I'm a shadow of my real self." There was a time, for both of us, when the future held promises instead of threats.

We laugh.

Oh, it's good to laugh.

We hang up because her younger son has come home from school and is lying on the floor again, sobbing. Francie must go now. She knows how to give strength to the child.

We all do.

We know how to support our husbands, too.

The problem is ourselves.

Who's helping us?

We're helping each other.

*Mainstay* isn't about dying; it's about living married to someone sick — not through a short fatal cancer or heart attack but through years and years of illness without cure. There may be seven million of us well spouses on this path, men as well as women. All we usually see of each other is a vanishing heel or an occasional, distant wave. In this book, we will finally get together. We'll tell each other our stories and share our hard-won learning, along with practical, workable advice — some of it from professionals in various fields but most of it from the common personal experience of the real experts, those of us who live here.

You're not alone.

# Mainstay

# Chapter 1
# Something Is Wrong

"I'll call as soon as I hear." Ted spoke calmly so as not to alert the children. He pulled me close, smelling sweet at the neck. Then he took Seth's hand and the two of them walked out the door toward the elevator. Everything looked okay: a tall, curly-haired man with his tall, curly-haired son. Nobody would have noticed that the man's stride fell slightly off, that his right foot failed to swing forward as surely as his left.

"Come on, keed!" I whispered to Debbie, whose tie-dyed shirt looked more dirty than dyed and whose gold-rimmed granny glasses sat funny on her nose. They were always getting twisted and after I'd straightened them out with the special pliers and stuck them into the straight black hair behind her ears, we grabbed hands and ran to the elevator. The whole family wore glasses. Whenever we boarded a bus together, people would stare us to our seats, figuring the genetic possibilities. "It's okay," I always wanted to call out, "we're just readers."

The tar of 86th Street on New York's Upper West Side was already soft under my sandals. We were medium-sized and loose-jointed and straight-haired together, Debbie and I.

"You put your face in the water last night?" I'd been so worried about Ted, I'd forgotten the basic daily worries.

"Kind of." Debbie's sneaker laces flopped as she walked straight ahead, considering. She practiced for her daily swim at night in the safety of the family tub. "Imaginative and artistic," her camp counselor reported. "She'll swim when she's ready." I wanted to help her more, but I couldn't keep my mind on much. I mustn't call Ted at the office. We had to keep the line open.

"Bye bye!" I waved at her sweet face in the big yellow camp bus — windows open, kids' arms on the sills, everything normal. Wasn't it?

Hurry back. He could know already. He could be calling you. Let it be no. But if it's yes, it would explain so much: I had begun to look back and pinpoint strange moments in our dozen years together.

No phone was ringing in the quiet, dark apartment. I made iced tea in the red-tiled kitchen from which I'd masterminded so many messy birthday parties and all those overly ambitious dinners we used to turn out when we still ate chicken Kiev and steak au poivre. I carried the cold glass through the swinging door into the dim, high-ceiled dining room. In the center stood the round oak table I'd bought in Greenwich Village on my twenty-eighth birthday when it seemed I'd never get married. Our blue Portuguese plates rested on the ledge of paneling that ran around the room. Ted had brought them home one day shortly after the wedding.

I sat at my desk. From this heap of tabletop and file cabinets, I'd managed — amidst diapers and unraveling buttonholes — to launch a writing career. I'd won a national grant, appeared on radio and, once, even seen my face before me on that temporary veil of immortality, television. I was living out the life dream. Mine, after all, were simple goals: a happy marriage, children wiser than I, plus a small contribution to the world of letters — none of your sailboats, none of your senate seats. Yet, working part-time, I could barely haul in enough dollars to pay for the kids' private school, and their camps, and the psychiatrist — all that took about twelve thousand dollars. That day in August 1977, I was working on the dregs, an encyclopedia piece presenting the history of the adhesive bandage.

Appropriate.

By noon, we'd know. The doctor was leaving for vacation at noon and nothing alters a doctor's vacation plans.

Ted must be sitting at his desk in midtown Manhattan,

staring at picture layouts. Passersby might not see him raise his light, changeable eyes today, might not feel the generous approval that usually radiated from his lean face. He liked to shore folks up. That's one reason I married him.

EDITORS TO WED, some young headline writer had slapped atop our small announcement in the *Times*. It had taken us years to find each other: we'd married only after spending our twenties fine-tuning ourselves into people somewhat different from those our parents, in the way of parents, had labored to produce. After the ceremony, we bumped across the water in a speedboat to Fire Island and paraded around a damp, gritty cottage laughing and grilling our first "married" cheese sandwiches. Ted walked around in sandals looking wonderfully Mediterranean, and I wore my tight white jeans that the men standing in doorways on Upper Broadway had always applauded.

At last we'd caught up with our friends. We were getting ours. This was life and we were living it. What did we care if skies were gray that first day? We walked on the beach in the mist, Ted's arm around my shoulder and my hand in his hip pocket so I could feel more of his body as he walked. We saw brightness ahead. We'd both crossed out so many unwanted possibilities in our twenties that we knew exactly what we did want in the future: each other, children, work, travel. And we wanted a marriage in which we both felt like equal partners. We'd each paid homage to an older sibling and neither of us ever wanted to feel like the smaller or weaker part of a twosome again.

"Ireland, we'll walk around it." Ted's stride in the cold sand lasted longer than mine. "When we're old and the kids have gone to college, I'll show you everything."

"Greece." I tried to walk at my own pace without exactly slowing Ted down. "Egypt."

"Jews don't go to Egypt so much lately."

"Oh. I forgot. Ireland, then. Greece." It was good that Ted was a Jew. He could have those warm Mediterranean rages of his, slamming doors and giving me what for and then breaking the ice and making up. They'd make the perfect balance for my Yankee silences, stony and treacherous. Monday morning we started home.

My wedding ring looked so bright in the speedboat and on the train and in the subway. One day it would look worn. By then we'd have raised two or three children and published twenty-five books, seventeen for Ted and eight for me. We'd appear in *Who's Who*. I'd be the first woman in my family to . . .

"Wait a sec." Ted put down the suitcase as we stepped out of the subway. "I've got to rest a minute."

Rest? Strange. I stood next to the stairs without touching the wall. Maybe it was his rheumatic heart?

Nine-thirty.

I couldn't get going on the history of the bandage. I stood up from my desk and went into the bedroom to straighten out the cheap old green and white madras spread we loved. I kicked the green and yellow Greek rug into place and pulled at the gauzy white curtains that blew in at the slightest disturbance of air. From the street came the smell of tomato sauce. New York seems so Spanish, so Middle Eastern, so Mediterranean in summer. We'd taken our first trip shortly after we were married. In Mykonos Ted knew so much! How to call for room service in Greek as the sun fell smack into the sea. What armies had passed through what brown plains. And then we got to Delphi.

"You're too energetic," Ted remarked as we fell into bed that night, his new beard prickly and endearing. "You walk too fast."

Was something wrong with that rheumatic heart of his?

In Cyprus it was raining. Ted stretched out on the double bed, his long legs touching the wall, and pulled the sheet up over his ear.

"I don't know what's wrong. I'm just tired. I think I need to rest."

"Okay." I walked too fast. I planned too much. And I hated shopping. Ted loved shopping. I'd shop, then.

In a corner store that sold magazines, I found some comic books written in Greek. Should I buy *Herakles*? Would he think it was a dig? But it was perfect, a real classic comic.

"Now that's what I call a classic comic!" Ted laughed and sat up while I turned on the light. His long, handsome face the same, the curly hair matted against the side, the light eyes pleased.

"Everything will be all right, won't it? When we get home?" I stood beside the bed in my white jeans, remembering centuries of advice on marriage.

"Everything's fine right now." He swung his long legs down and reached for his shirt. "Let's go. We'll order boiled beef in British accents."

Back home we marched against Vietnam down Fifth Avenue but we avoided Sixth when the Beatles drew crowds there at lunchtime. We were happy to stay home and be grown-ups under the madras spread, or out in Riverside Park reading the *Times* on a Sunday, or at the movie houses on Upper Broadway — each other's permanent date.

"Congratulations, sir." I toasted him at the French restaurant when he got promoted.

"Congratulations, madame." He held my hand by the bed at New York Hospital. "The kid is wiped out but you don't even look tired."

Nine forty-five.

I walked into Seth's room, full of baseball cards and toy soldiers arranged in fighting patterns on the lower bunk in front of the red, white, and blue American flag quilt my mother had knitted for him. At night he climbed up into Space Ship Greenstein in the upper bunk. There were portholes in its guardrail and through one stuck the muzzle of a plastic gun. His transparent boxes stood fogged and dented in their rows on the windowsill, displaying his extravagantly categorized objects. "He's the only kid that loves to put the toys back on their shelves!" his nursery teacher had exclaimed years ago. I'd expected her to comment on his interest in square roots. "He's quiet," she went on. "And shows some immaturity of temper." "He's only four," I replied. Taken aback, I forgot to mention he could read. Ten years old and turning into a smaller version of Ted — beginning to lengthen out, his hair once soft and fine grown curly, his face taking on the same deadpan look Ted's offered: a look saying, go on, kid me. I won't let on I know and that will make it all the funnier.

What a winter we had passed through. Seth had caught strep and taken antibiotics. At a routine visit to the pediatrician, he'd troubled her with a strange heartbeat. Did he have a heart murmur like Ted's? The bad kind? She arranged an electrocardiogram. "I don't want a ba-ad heart," Seth had said, folding his long-legged self into a corner of the lower bunk afterward, as his face undid into tears. "Oh, sweetheart." I held him close and started to tell him he didn't have any such thing. But how did I know? Something broke in me, sitting on that bunk. It felt as if an elastic band had pulled too far. As soon as we found out Seth was okay, we started worrying about Debbie's eyes.

I left Seth's room and walked into Debbie's. Here light filtered through the blue and white checkered curtains onto the spew of plastic toys, dolls, paints, and dress-up clothes. She had watched her twisting mobile so intently in her first months of life, although her eyes were very crossed.

"Watch her now," I'd told the pediatrician at Debbie's second or third checkup. "She's smiling. But it's at my voice. Is she blind?" The pediatrician had snapped on her flashlight. "She's got the light reflex, all right." She snapped it off. "But I won't know until she's six months old whether she can see."

We weren't too scared. Ted's eyes had been crossed at birth, too, and surgery had fixed his. Or almost — one eye saw better far and the other near, and he'd had a lot of trouble hitting baseballs.

We knew before six months that Debbie could see, and at one year she'd had two eye muscles surgically relocated. I'd surprised myself by praying throughout the two-hour operation. After Seth's heart murmur threat, her ophthalmologist left New York. The new one demanded a second, sudden surgery. During that four-hour operation at Christmastime, I couldn't pray. It was entirely gone. Instead, I played with a ball of plastic dough for four straight hours and could barely move my hands when she was wheeled back, a small white lump on a dolly cart.

Ten o'clock.

In the high-ceiled living room, Ted's more formal desk sat as near the window as he could get it. He'd always found this apartment too dark. Above the desk hung the cowboy piñata he'd brought back from a conference in Mexico. That was the year he'd been made a vice president. "Every step up in publishing takes you further from writing," he said that night as we sat on the dark couch my mother had given us when she moved. Sundays the kids and I removed to playground or museum while Ted sat at his desk. Here he'd written a picture history of Spain. Then a full history of Athens. Now his desk supported a stack of research books for a history of Greece during World War II. The piñata swung in a slow circle, papier-mâché horse with papier-mâché Lone Ranger with papier-mâché hat — it fell off all the time — and ribbon after ribbon of yellow crepe paper, for the horse's withers.

Exactly the soft yellow I'd painted with the fine brush into the recessed niches between the room's fancy panelings. Ted had stood on a ladder that summer night in shorts and bare chest spattering oil-based white to roll the ceiling, singing *Oy, how I love to be a peyntor* in a Yiddish accent. The paint brought a beautiful white glow into the room filled with dark furniture from the Salvation Army. So after a late start, we had it all: careers, kids, marriage. There was just one problem.

Ted was experiencing some episodes of impotence. Of course we'd seen a therapist. In the '60s and '70s, everything was psychological and, therefore, curable. Change required only right thought, right action. These could be found via one Dr. Miller. We'd been seeing him anyway for general angst: everybody in Manhattan's upwardly mobile professional class saw a psychiatrist in those days.

Clearly, said Dr. Miller, Ted was anxious. Clearly Maggie should learn to belly dance, buy a vibrator, turn down the lights, shop for lingerie at Bonwit's, cook even more gourmet, and puff the pillows up in satin pillowcases. "Be more of a woman," one of Dr. Miller's therapy group members instructed me, repeating an advertising slogan of the day, "and he'll be more of a man."

I found myself profoundly offended.

In vain did I describe the delicacy of sympathies that binds two people — these were Me-Decade swingers. So I kept quiet and grew my hair longer. I wore more jewelry. I painted my nails a brighter red. I went around without a bra. But often, when we got into bed, forget it.

"His penis," I said to my group, thinking I'd observed something that might be useful, "is cooler to the touch than you'd expect. What do you think that could mean?"

"Oh, my God!" they said. "How castrating!"

A simple question. Temperature had seemed to offer a clue. But I learned not to ask any more questions. Oh, it wasn't at all funny. It was extremely sad. Everything was so good except the one thing. I had never expected to have this much or *this little*.

Most women know how to take the heat off a man for life's occasional impotences, how to reassure, comfort. But what happens if impotence continues to surface unpredictably? One day at our joint session with Dr. Miller, Ted and I asked him to put us into the new sex therapy we'd read about — the Masters and Johnson program.

Beautiful Dr. Jasonson took us step by step through the program, even though Ted's skin felt funny and uncomfortable with her recommended nonsexual strokings and even though I found step-by-step sex only slightly less mechanized than vibrator sex. "Creepy," Ted described to her the sensation on the skin of his thighs, "pre-itchy."

"That's anxiety," Dr. Jasonson informed him.

I sure liked Dr. Jasonson. She understood the pressures of raising two kids in Manhattan. She believed the husband should take equal responsibility with the wife in the home. Ted believed it, too. Or had said so, back before we married, before the kids were born. Somehow it wasn't working out. Dr. Jasonson explained to Ted why it was natural for me to be angry if he went to bed after the party and didn't help with the dishes. "Even if you were tired," Dr. Jasonson went on, "don't you think Maggie was tired, too?" When she said it, it seemed so reasonable. When I said it I waited too long and then got too mad and then Ted would get mad back and slam the bedroom door and the beautiful Greek tiles showing red ships on the green-blue sea would fall off the wall and break. I was extra devastated when Dr. Jasonson turned us back to Dr. Miller uncured.

What was wrong? I'd been subtly programmed not to discuss sex with Dr. Miller, so I concentrated on the unfair division of labor.

"He won't move the air conditioner," I told Dr. Miller in my private session. "He says it's too heavy. Maybe it's his heart murmur? His parents never let him lift a finger, pack a car, or move anything heavy, so maybe he's just used to not doing stuff. Or maybe I'm making an unreasonable demand?"

"No," Dr. Miller gave one of his rare replies from the Naugahyde throne, "I move my air conditioner. But take the pressure off him. Hire someone."

Many of Dr. Miller's solutions involved the expenditure of money, dollars that I had to go out and earn since we'd agreed my free-lance income would fill any gap.

Alone, Ted and I worked out a sexual life, better than we had through either groupies or doctors. And as a family we had lovely times. Ted suggested a series of little Saturday bus trips into the wilds of New Jersey or around Manhattan by boat. We took the Staten Island Ferry, the wind blowing Seth's curly hair into a part and raising Debbie's soft black hair straight up. "The Greensteins at Bay" we'd captioned the photo a fellow passenger had taken — Ted and I stood front to front with our arms around each other and our faces turned, beaming, into the camera. You can tell the '60s are over because my Sassoon haircut is gone and I've got the long smooth brown hair you nurse along until forty.

"Out! Out! Brief bear!" Ted would exorcise the nightly bear from Seth's bedroom. The two of them would go off to the park Saturdays with a baseball and bat, since Ted was determined that Seth would never suffer the humiliation he'd known as a kid from being unable to hit a ball.

"Are you available for tea?" he inquired of Debbie one Saturday, and took her off to where Eloise drank hers — the Plaza Hotel. They rode up and down in the elevators, looking for the floors on Eloise's map. Debbie borrowed my scarf and knotted it just where I knot it.

So Ted and I would smile at each other over the children's heads and rejoice in the long-limbed, faulty-visioned family we had created. One sunny Saturday we took the bus to a park full of irises in New Jersey. We kicked a soccer ball around and then fell onto the soft cut grass: the Greensteins at Play. No life is perfect. Marriage has its stages. We loved each other. Everything would be all right. One day we'd have the agents and the editors we needed and we'd move out to the country to a big old house and the kids could have a dog. "Smile," Ted said as he held the camera to his eye. But his photographs, once sharp and finely focused, began to turn out blurry.

Whenever I got trapped into mentioning any of my problems with Ted in therapy, my groupies would instruct me to shape up and get out of the marriage. Once in a while I would wonder if maybe they were right. But the kids were too young. Maybe when they reached eight and ten? But surely things would be better by then, if we just tried a little harder? Of course, things were getting better all the time! And Ted wasn't an irresponsible man.

Was he?

The telephone by our bed stopped working. Ted promised to

take it in for repair since the shop was only a block from his office. "You did promise," I reminded him occasionally, trying not to nag because the last thing I ever wanted to become was a nag. A year or so later when I reminded him, he shouted from his desk in the living room. "If you want it done so much, do it yourself!"

He seemed to be getting angry.

One day in the foyer by the door I asked him to mail a single business letter of mine on his way to work. It was snowing out and rotten cold and one of the kids was sick.

"No," he said, crossing the hall in his business suit and tie and coat. "It's too heavy."

"Too heavy? For Pete's sake, it would fit in your jacket pocket!"

That time, I slammed the door. When he was gone, I got out the yellow pages. I actually looked up divorce lawyers. I stared at their names. I didn't believe in divorce. The kids were too young. Besides, Ted loved them. They loved Ted. Ted and I loved each other. People often told us we were the only couple they knew who seemed to get along. We were the model. When we came into a room together we turned a corner into a curve, someone said. If this one or that one could just have a marriage like ours. . . . Ted and I would smile at each other. Despite everything, we did love each other. We just had some trouble now and then getting through our anniversary dinners. But isn't that what all the cartoons are about?

In 1976, when the kids turned seven and nine, we vacationed on Cape Cod. They ran in great looping circles on the beach, Seth cautious in his nearsightedness and Debbie recklessly happy to be freed of first grade. I ran beside them. Ted stood alone by the water with his hands pulling down at the pockets of his windbreaker, a long-legged bird. "We could save money," he said as I approached, "and buy a summer place."

Save money? I couldn't work fast enough to pay the four thousand we owed Dr. Miller.

"How can you run like that?" Ted squinted from the noon sun. "Don't you get tired?"

"No," I said, stopping suddenly. "Do you?"

"Lately, I get out of breath."

"What do you mean?"

He undid his long stride and ran a very short distance and back.

"See, I can't . . . breathe enough." His face looked distant, as if calculating something on the inside.

"Is it your heart?" Behind me, the sound of the surf; above, the sky dark with too much sun.

"No. It's more, maybe . . . my lungs? I'd better go for a checkup when we get back."

The doctor said Ted was in great shape — hadn't gained a pound since college. Throughout the winter, Ted seemed withdrawn and sad.

"Are you mad at me?" I felt guilty all the time.

"It's the office." Ted stood by the window in the living room, his long fingers knotted behind his back. His publishing house had changed ownership and all the editors were being instructed to bring in a net income equal to eleven times their own salaries. "I don't know if I can make my quota." He looked thinner and tired and worried. "I'm afraid I might lose my job."

"Oh, don't be dumb! You're a vice president!" I was working on venting, letting it all hang out.

That winter, after Debbie's Christmas surgery, Ted walked into a glass door.

He bumped into the couch and broke his toe.

Leaning over a drinking fountain at work, he couldn't swallow correctly and began to choke. Dying? He couldn't breathe. Was this dying?

He got the flu. A funny sensation ringed his kneecaps.

"I call it hot kneecaps," he explained cheerily from under the madras spread. "It's the same as that creepy flesh I get on my thighs."

When we walked a few blocks to the movies, his feet seemed to hesitate like an old man's, the right foot to swing forward more slowly. It made me impatient, annoyed.

At home he talked in a slower, sometimes repetitive manner. It drove me wild.

And he never wanted to go anywhere anymore. He took to bed earlier and earlier.

In April we attended my high school's twenty-fifth reunion and Ted fell down and sprained an ankle. Using crutches exhausted him. Again, he had no breath. He went for a second physical. "Congratulations," the doctors cheered again. "You are in perfect health."

In May he began to have trouble urinating.

In June, Debbie turned eight, her black hair shining, her eyes straighter than ever behind her glasses, and she'd come out of the dip she took at school after her Christmas operation. Seth would turn ten in August. Ten and eight. The smallest sheep over the stile. This was the summer. Should I leave Ted? There were so many and such constant choices during the Me Decade. They wore a person out. And since everything was psychologically based, a person might not suspect that something could be terribly, physically wrong.

"They took it! They took it!" Later in June, Ted's book on Greece during the war was accepted by his favorite publishing house. This was the break he'd been waiting for. Saved by the bell. Sooner or later he could quit his job and write full-time. We would laugh and love!

"It's wonderful." Our friends Sid and Mim raised glasses of champagne to Ted on their patio high over the Hudson. Oh, everything was going to be all right.

"Terrific. I see you guys surrounded by green leaves in a country house," our Wall Street friend Stan prophesied at a Lebanese restaurant to which Ted had pushed him in his wheelchair. In their senior year at Harvard, Stan had turned a convertible over on himself, but there we were in our early forties and everything else was going to be fine.

In July the left side of Ted's tongue went numb.

"Maybe it's something wrong with a tooth," I suggested.

Our dentist urged him to see a neurologist. A couple of days before the appointment, the whole left side of his face went not exactly numb, but "creepy," the way his thighs and knees had felt.

"Maybe it's a pinched nerve," Ted suggested as we waited day by day for the appointment.

"I drew a picture of myself today," Debbie said at the dining table, her glasses funny again. "I lay down on a piece of paper and drew —"

"I played second base," Seth said, the sweat that had rolled down his neck during the sun of the day marking rivulets of dirt on his camp shirt. You could see the strong sinews of the muscles in his slender pitching arm. "And I hit a grounder. . . ."

They didn't get much attention as we waited.

Ted looked worn the July evening he returned from the neurologist. The children jumped up from the table to greet him and he staggered under their welcome. When the kids were watching TV, Ted came into the kitchen to give me the full report. "I have to go into a hospital for tests."

I leaned over the dishwasher's throbbing surface for comfort. "What are they testing for?"

"A possible neurological disorder." Ted took off his tie. "Maybe a spinal infection." He looked absent as he unbuttoned the top of his blue shirt. "A spinal tap. Yes, that's the name of it."

A spinal tap. I could hear the water dripping in the sink. "What are you most afraid of?"

"A brain tumor." His face looked like Seth's when he'd been scared of a bad heart.

"Oh, honey." I stood up and put my arms around him. "That couldn't be." A brain tumor couldn't be, could it? We stood silently, while outside, car horns punctuated the summer traffic.

When Debbie was lying between her Snoopy sheets and Seth sailing through the sky in his upper bunk and Ted pretending to watch the late news, I walked to my desk. I took up my medical dictionary and turned to "spinal tap." These, I read, are used to test for meningitis, brain tumor, and multiple sclerosis. I turned to "brain tumor." Well, Ted would be much relieved. Headaches he didn't have, nor convulsions, nor nausea. Could you call his walking into the glass door a vision disturbance? No, it wasn't a tumor. Good. I turned to "meningitis." He had no fever and no stiff neck. I turned to "multiple sclerosis."

In a single paragraph I read about numbness in cheek and tongue, about changes in gait, about problems with urination, about slurring of speech and problems with swallowing, about blurred vision, about extreme responsiveness to weather and temperature, about weakness, fatigue, and loss of strength, and about impotence — one of the very earliest signs, often appearing many years before diagnosis.

"Ted!" I called out. In those last seconds of my innocence, I didn't want to know anything Ted didn't know. As he came into the room, I whispered, "Here, you'd better take a look at this."

Eleven. Why didn't Ted call me?

I got up from my desk and made more iced tea. I stood at the kitchen window looking into the narrow space between the back of our building and the front. Once I'd been standing here and flames from a fire several stories up had shot down, orange flames with black smoke, real flames, real smoke, not something on TV.

"Multiple sclerosis would explain so much," I'd ventured to Dr. Miller. "Maybe even the impotence?"

"No, no," he'd said, in his office high over Park Avenue. "Nothing like impotence would show up so fast."

"It says so in the book."

"No. I've told you. No." He stirred not on his throne. Case closed.

But on the slight possibility that Ted might be sick with something, we should act fast. We should, Dr. Miller instructed, get ourselves a big disability policy from a private insurance company.

Multiple sclerosis? I stood at my kitchen window and called up all the cases of multiple sclerosis I'd ever known. My parents' friend, a dancer. Her husband massaged her seventy-pound body daily. "Doesn't she look great today?" he would say as he wheeled her into our house. "Isn't she a miracle?" Her leg spasmed and clattered on the footrest. It was not a teenager's idea of miracle.

In college I took a train through whirling snow to St. Paul, where my parents had temporarily relocated. They deposited me promptly at the church's Young People's Group. All the kids were tall and blond and believed in the resurrection of the body. Except for me and Bernard. He sat in a wheelchair and was majoring in biology in hopes of finding a cure for his multiple sclerosis before it killed him. In January we wrote letters to each other. He sent a picture of himself that didn't show the chair. After an evening of inner turmoil in my eastern dormitory, I convinced myself that I didn't have to love Bernard just because he was sick, just because he could be the lame and the halt and the blind wrapped into one and I ought to.

My mother's college friend had gotten multiple sclerosis just before her wedding. In later years her husband would walk home from work at noon to turn her over in her bed so she wouldn't get bedsores.

It can't be that.

This can't be happening to us.

If it was, I would never leave Ted. He shouldn't have to face that horror alone. If it was multiple sclerosis, so much would be clarified. Our problems wouldn't be Ted's fault. They would be the illness's. I would have married the man I'd thought I was marrying. The changes in Ted would be only the illness. I'd make up for it. I'd make up for everything. Ted would never become a vegetable to be turned over at noon.

Quarter of twelve!

I walked a nervous circle in the kitchen. When we'd painted this room a glossy white, Ted had stopped after supper because he felt too tired. Angrily, I'd worked to midnight to finish. No more anger. Not now. "Sure sounds like it," he'd said the night I showed him the encyclopedia. "But I don't think it is. I think it's a brain tumor."

The next night at supper he'd told the kids he was going into the hospital to find out why he'd been having trouble balancing.

They looked blank over their hamburgers.

"Have you noticed Daddy's been walking a little funny since this spring when he sprained his ankle?"

"No," they both said.

"Well, maybe a little," Debbie added, looking up at Ted, considering.

Seth put his hamburger roll down on his blue and white plate and didn't say anything at all.

Ted and I took a cab to the hospital the morning before Seth's tenth birthday. I carried the suitcase, trying to make it look sporty, casual. I tried not to think, "This may be just the first time I carry the suitcase." The nurses put Ted into a wheelchair against his will, as he tried not to think, "Maybe I'll end up in one of these." At the teller's window, I slipped two thin thousand-dollar bills (the first I'd ever seen!) under the wire. It was the kids' school payment for September, but Dr. Miller had warned us to pay cash. That way nothing would show on our Blue Cross bill, and if you held your private disability insurance for two years without making a single claim, he said, they could never disqualify you. Ted settled in a bed between a boy with a spinal injury like Stan's and a man with a brain tumor.

"I'm safe now," Ted said softly into my ear as I bent to kiss him goodnight. "They've already given out the tumor to this room." His breath smelled as sweet as ever.

I took the bus home to get up Seth's birthday party. I let him open his Asterix comic and his James Bond car that night because it seemed so lonely without Ted.

The next morning, when I walked into Ted's room, the curtain was drawn ominously around his bed. A doctor sat by the bed holding a long needle: I'd heard that any wrong move, any nick, during a spinal tap could paralyze a person forever. The phone rang. Ted's parents had called Seth to wish him a happy birthday and he'd told them Daddy was in the hospital. I'd thought of everything but that!

The morning after that I found myself back behind the curtain meeting Ted's neurologist. His mustache was much too neat.

"We don't have an answer yet," Dr. Astor said. "There'll be a few more tests. It'll take about two weeks to collate results. I'll call you that Tuesday morning. I go on vacation at noon."

"Is multiple sclerosis one of the things you're testing for?" I asked it straight out.

"Yes. That, and spinal infection. But," he cleared his throat, "we call it a neuromuscular disorder." He turned to leave.

He couldn't even say the words!

"They ruled out tumor." Ted's voice against the pillows sounded cheerful and distant.

I left.

Fifteen ten-year-old boys were coming for lunch.

Five of twelve.

The instant the phone rang, I slammed down my glass and ran through the swinging door to the dining room.

"Hi." Ted's voice sounded normal.

"What did he say?" I sat down fast.

"He hasn't even called! The damn phone hasn't rung all

morning. I've been sitting at my desk until just a minute ago when I left to go to the bathroom. He didn't call there while I was gone, did he?"

"Nope."

"Okay. Let's hang up."

We were entirely together.

Two of twelve. It rang again.

I didn't want to know anymore. I wanted to sit straight up in that desk chair forever.

"Hi," I said, warm, close, there for Ted.

"This is Dr. Astor," a tense voice reported. "I've been trying steadily since 10 A.M. to reach your husband at his office, Mrs. Greenstein. But either his line is busy or he doesn't answer, so I'm calling you. The report is affirmative. The lab has put together the cell counts for the spinal tap with the other physiological signs and has come up with a diagnosis of possible neuromuscular disorder."

"Do you mean multiple sclerosis?"

"You could call it that, Mrs. Greenstein, but we don't."

"But that's what you mean?"

"Now, don't get excited. It's not definite. You can only really be one hundred percent sure after watching it for a year. So, I'd say it's ninety percent sure. And besides, you're lucky. There is a lot of research going on now, a lot of money going into neuromuscular disorders. We're at the point of a breakthrough. Could be in a matter of years, months. So don't worry."

"Will you please call my —"

He'd hung up.

Ted. Oh, Ted. My poor Ted.

I would have to tell him?

That bastard! Dr. Astor was actually making me tell Ted! It should be the other way around! Ted should be telling me!

"Well, I knew it all the time," Ted replied in a clear voice.

"You didn't think it was a tumor?"

"No. I knew. I'm going to ring him now," Ted added, his competent managerial self. "I need to find out what to do."

"Yes. Call me back."

I waited. I would take care of Ted. He would be happy. I would make everything right. I would fix it. How could I find a fifty-thousand-dollar-a-year job? I'd start looking tomorrow.

When he called back in a few minutes, his voice sounded hurt. "It rang ten times," he said, smaller, less powerful. "A service finally answered. 'Dr. Astor is not available,' " he imitated the woman's voice. " 'Dr. Astor has left for the airport —' " His voice came to a stop and I knew he could no longer control it.

"Honey," I began, as the solid ground beneath us turned to quicksand. It was not only that Ted would suffer, and that our future and the children's had suddenly vanished. It was also that we were no longer equal: Dr. Astor had made that quite clear.

# Chapter 2
# Getting the News

News is whatever changes the future. Bad news threatens it. Ancient kings occasionally killed the bringers of bad news. No wonder doctors hesitate to deliver it. Yet thousands of people get the news of chronic illness every week — as do their wives or husbands, their children, their parents, and their friends. Sometimes the news is abrupt and stunning; sometimes suspicion has been slowly gathering so that the words "You're sick" bring a kind of relief.

When people think "sick" they tend to imagine a man who falls to the pavement with a heart attack or a woman who finds the wrong kind of lump in her breast. This is acute illness. You get better. Or you die. Acute illness is entirely alarming and absorbing and it's relatively — a year or maybe twice that — short. Our medicine concerns itself mainly with acute illness because doctors and drugs can often do something about it. They can cure it. Chronic illnesses are just that: chronic, incurable. You don't get better. Nobody wants to deal with them, not even doctors.

Chronic illnesses don't always kill, or not for decades. They limit and disable. They blind. They bring pain. They threaten adulthood or sexuality. They age, robbing the sickest of energy for anything but biological functioning. They paralyze and leave the brain alert or they snuff out memory and logic and leave the body robust. But they don't go away.

How many Americans suffer from chronic illness? Perhaps

twenty to twenty-five million. Loose estimates prevail because it's hard to distinguish mild cases from severe. For example, over twenty-two million Americans suffer from chronic obstructive pulmonary disease (emphysema and bronchitis) and/or its close relative, asthma. This three-part syndrome accounts for more lost workdays than any other illness. Yet it's impossible to really know how many of those twenty-two million who have trouble breathing find their lives substantially modified daily and year after year.

The National Center for Health Statistics tries to get a general idea. Each year it surveys noninstitutionalized chronically ill civilians. "For 1985 we estimate 9,044,000 people disabled enough so that they cannot carry on the major activity appropriate to their age level, be it student or homemaker or employed worker," reports Sandy Smith, chief of information at the center. "Another 13,228,000 were disabled to the point that they must modify their major activity, reducing or changing their work in some manner." Confusingly, that's twenty-two-plus million people again — yet these aren't the same twenty-two million who have trouble breathing. These are the hard-core chronically ill.

Another way to get a grasp on numbers and on the problems of distinguishing this from that is to put together the totals of the sick as estimated by various national organizations (see Appendix A) that correlate information relevant to specific illnesses. Here are some estimates for 1985:

| | |
|---|---|
| COPD plus asthma | 22,305,000 |
| Rheumatoid arthritis | 7,000,000 |
| Diabetes | 5,800,000 |
| Cancer | 5,000,000 |
| Coronary heart disease | 4,670,000 |
| Alzheimer's and related disorders | 2,500,000 |
| Stroke | 1,900,000 |
| Parkinson's disease | 1,000,000 |
| Lupus | 500,000 |
| Multiple sclerosis | 250,000 |
| Myasthenia gravis | 100,000 |
| Kidney disease, dialysis | 85,000 |
| Postpolio syndrome | 75,000 |

That's more than fifty-one million people, but plenty of men and women with diabetes or rheumatoid arthritis or asthma, for example, proceed with their expected lives and their work. We can't distinguish the severely from the mildly impaired. And not all of these fifty-one million are suffering from truly chronic conditions. The five million Americans listed with cancer, for instance, didn't all have cancer in 1985. Some three million of these were considered cured by then because they had passed a five-year mark without recurrence. Of the two million cancer cases remaining on the books in 1985, half were expected to die within five years — the other half to be cured. Cancer doesn't count as a true chronic illness.

Nor, necessarily, do the heart conditions. Cardiologists can't give the clear-cut, five-year plans oncologists do. Full or partial recovery has come to some of those four and a half million living Americans who'd had coronaries by the end of 1985. Death has come to others. And some of the nearly two million with strokes are getting better today, instead of worse.

And yet acute illnesses may drag on sufficiently to feel chronic — the slower leukemias or Hodgkin's disease come to mind. To further complicate the picture, chronic illnesses may possess acute phases. This overlap helps account for why it's hard to come by a solid number of the chronically ill. Does it matter to the reader? The definition is foggy and will remain foggy. If the shoe fits, it's yours.

You are the well spouse. How many wives and husbands of those twenty-two million sick enough to give up or alter their work could there be? Here we move into wilder surmise. About six million are under eighteen. That brings us right down to sixteen million. If they have married at a rate commensurate with the rest of the nation's adults, roughly ten million would have husbands and wives. (In 1984, 65.8 percent of males over eighteen were married and 60.8 percent of females.) Are there ten million well spouses? Anecdotal evidence suggests that the chronically ill divorce more frequently. Perhaps they marry less frequently. Sometimes the well spouses become sick them selves. Would you believe a minimum of seven million well spouses?

That's twice as many as belong to the National Rifle Association. Do we have a lobby?

No, the well spouses of the chronically ill are barely defined, barely studied. Few people know who we are or what we need.

When the well spouse turns to authorities, she may even find the enemy. Doctors and nurses often instruct us in how to make the patient's life easier. Psychotherapists detail the patient's fears. Physiotherapists explain how to move a patient's ankle or an elbow painlessly. But for us? *Nada.* We don't have a name. We don't even know our own needs.

This book attempts to give us well spouses a name and a consciousness of each other by describing our lives. We must become our own authorities. We will focus on spouses in their young adulthood or in early middle age. In those age brackets, illness comes as a surprise. Yet the shoe fits all ages.

Many of the psychologists and therapists who speak in these pages have themselves dealt with a chronic illness at home. You can often tell them from those who haven't by the tendency of the latter to dwell on expressing emotions and of the former to mention getting away for a break.

Well, then, what is the life of the well spouse?

It starts when you get the news.

In Houston, a couple in their late thirties finds out that one of them has amylateral sclerosis, or Lou Gehrig's disease. This cripples and kills, usually in three years.

> The doctor told my wife first, then he told us both together. I'd been noticing slight differences that my wife was denying — tiredness, favoring of one leg. I was shocked. My wife was emotionally down for a day or so, but she decided early on she wouldn't learn about it. I read everything ever published. I talked a lot to doctors. It's not like other diseases. There's no treatment, no medication. There is nothing they can do. As we left, we asked when to make our next appointment. The doctor said, "Don't bother."
>
> I was just overcome with grief.

It's Lisa who's sick, although it's hard to tell from Tom's report. The illness has happened to both of them. Yet they adopted different behaviors upon the impact of the news. In its three-year life expectancy, their illness stands between the acute and the chronic. ALS is short enough so that by the time you recover from the news, it's almost time to move into the crisis of dying.

In Pasadena, Francie recalls getting the news of a fast-onset but treatable illness:

> When they told us kidney failure, I didn't know what they were talking about. Eric had never been sick a day in his life. All of a sudden, he might die. Everything changed.
>
> We couldn't tell Paul. We'd just put him on the plane to go off to college for the first time. We wanted him to spend at least his first week at school without knowing how sick his father was. He deserved one last innocent week.

Well spouses who are parents care desperately about protecting their children from the disappearing future. And for good reason. Here's a grown woman recalling how she felt at sixteen when she got the news of her father's chronic and incurable Parkinson's disease:

> I was sixteen when I finally found out my father had Parkinson's. I was glad it wasn't a brain tumor. But as soon as my mother told me, I knew I was no longer protected. The future narrowed.

Stunned as you both are, you face the narrowed future together. Yet not quite together. Remember the first time you looked at the man or woman you loved asleep? You looked at that vulnerable face and knew you would protect it no matter what. That person was perfectly safe with you. The feeling was similar, perhaps, to when you first looked at your newborn child. You would take care of this child no matter what. When you get a diagnosis of chronic illness, some of that feeling returns. The two of you are divided by being in different states, and you, the well one, will take care of the other. Except you're married and you're supposed to be equal, your spouse is supposed to be protecting and caring for you equally. You lose your expected future, first, and then your marital equality.

What lies ahead? Before examining the sudden darkness after diagnosis, let's acknowledge two conditions where diagnosis brings a measure of relief. The first is loss of cerebral functioning. If your spouse has been going slowly crazy with an organic brain disorder such as Alzheimer's, or exhibiting a mental illness such as schizophrenia, you'll be not only horrified but also reassured. All those signs, all those signals, finally make sense. Something is wrong. It hasn't been your distortion. You are not insane. Lonely, forever isolated from your spouse, but not crazy.

The same goes for the person whose spouse has suffered sexual dysfunction. The list of illnesses that may produce altered sexual function in women or in men include diabetes, Parkinson's, MS, liver and kidney disease, and blood pressure and vessel diseases. Certain medications, sometimes including chemotherapy, also affect sexual functioning. Yet both man and wife may remain unenlightened as to why the couple is experiencing sexual trouble. Puzzlement and hurt turn to anger and accusation. Professionals may increase the puzzlement.

"It's not at all uncommon that couples affected by the male's chronic impotence are sent to psychologists or psychiatrists or sex counselors before discovering that the impotence has a medical cause," says Eileen MacKenzie, who with her husband, Bruce MacKenzie, founded IMPOTENTS ANONYMOUS (I.A. for Impotent Men and I-ANON for Partners of Impotent Men) in 1981 and the IMPOTENCE INSTITUTE OF AMERICA, INC., in 1983. "From 1983 through 1985," she reports, "we received over sixty thousand inquiries and about half of them tell that same story." This, despite the fact that conjecture over the cause of impotence has flipped since 1970 when 85 percent to 90 percent was considered psychologically based. Now it's the reverse — up to 65 percent or sometimes 80 percent is considered physiologically based.

The MacKenzies themselves went through the not uncommon experience, marrying after each had lost a spouse and then finding Bruce impotent. They went to a family doctor who knew Bruce had diabetes but who didn't even suggest his impotence might be physical. Instead the doctor gave the couple sexual counseling. When that didn't work, he sent them to sex therapists. When that didn't work, the therapists finally told Bruce to check in with a urologist. The urologist happened to specialize in impotence (only about one in three does) and found out that Bruce was 100 percent physically impotent from neuropathy caused by his diabetes.

"The experience of being impotent produces emotional stress to both man and wife," Eileen MacKenzie points out. "Women fear the man doesn't love them or they feel guilty because — whether they mean to or not — they get angry or upset at their impotent man and then feel guilty because they know he's a very good person."

Psychiatrist Domeena Renshaw, who directs the Loyola Sexual Dysfunction Clinic in Chicago, states (see Appendix B) that the wife of the impotent man is caught in a double bind. She can't win for losing. "If she approaches him for sex, she gets labeled demanding, domineering, and castrating. If she does not approach him, she is called infantile, passive, masochistic, nonsexual, or maternal." What's written about such wives is usually slanted in a sophisticated way to blame them for the problem. "There is always the implication that if the husband had a new partner who was more seductive or submissive or adoring or less maternal, he'd be fine."

Dr. Renshaw found that this isn't usually the case. In a study of 151 wives of men who had been impotent from eight months to twenty-one years, she found that only 32 could be described as angry, demanding, depreciating, and domineering. The majority, 119 wives, were found to be supportive, sensitive, and concerned. Fifty-seven of the men had turned to other women and 39 reported no change. Diagnosis relieves by taking the couple with illness-related sexual complications out of the fray of accusation and hurt.

Dr. John Rolland is one of those professionals who know personally the role of the well spouse. He was twenty-six and so was his wife when they heard she had metastatic cancer. A medical student, he took active care of her — bringing her home from hospitals to protect her from staph infections, drawing her blood himself.

"It was very hard," Dr. Rolland says, sitting in New Haven in the newly painted office of his recently founded Center for Illness in Families. Now in his mid-thirties, he recalls:

> The worst part was that we no longer shared a future. We didn't have children, or they would have provided a physical kind of future. Instead, our sense of time diverged. She lived day to day while I remained bound in a much longer future. I needed to study to get my medical degree. Then I needed to study for my psychiatric degree. I couldn't afford to get off that path by doing poorly in my studies. My future would be jeopardized.
>
> She was so young, yet she had no time. When she felt good, she wanted to go to Paris. She'd never seen Paris and once she

did fly over to visit. When she felt her sickest, it was just hours and days instead of weeks for her to think about. So we lived in a split frame, as far as time goes. And that really separates people.

She died at thirty, four years after diagnosis. He finished his studies and became a family therapist, opening the center in 1984. Here he and his colleagues counsel sick and well family members who are dealing with illness.

Effect on family life begins with the way a diagnosis is delivered. "The doctors," Dr. Rolland says, in his office full of warm, desert colors, "give a diagnosis but they frequently don't translate what it will mean into psychosocial terms for the family. Most don't have the training to do that." Because of this Dr. Rolland believes that when a family receives a diagnosis of chronic illness, they should be encouraged by their physicians to have a meeting with a mental health professional as part of the treatment plan. The professional could show the family how to understand and make use of its own coping resources. All families have strengths and weaknesses in how they cope. It helps to become aware of which is which in order to get ready to deal with a long illness. If a family needs more than a single session with a professional, they might seek short-term family therapy at the hospital or from a private therapist. Families needn't be pathological or neurotic to seek help. Most of the people Dr. Rolland sees aren't: "They're just ordinary people hit hard with hard news."

"The first five minutes of communication at the critical turning point of diagnosis can set up an emotional model for the whole course of the illness," Dr. Rolland continues in his office where plants absorb the light from small, high windows. "Who says what to whom matters a great deal. Whatever a doctor does at that vulnerable time can influence people for years. If he tells the news to the spouse first or gives the spouse different or harsher news than he gives the patient, he may not be just giving news. He may also be inadvertently implying 'You and I are in charge here. The patient is not in charge of himself any longer.' "

After diagnosis, families need information in order to proceed, in order to cope. With his combined medical and psychiatric training, Dr. Rolland provides a road map for each illness and some insight about itself to each family. Two things shape the new future: a family's style and which illness they must meet.

According to Dr. Rolland in "Toward a Psychosocial Typology of Chronic and Life-Threatening Illness" (see Appendix B), every illness raises four questions. How fast did it come on? Will it hold itself in abeyance, come in bouts, or simply worsen relentlessly? Will it be fatal? How disabling will it be? Let's take a brief look at Dr. Rolland's typology. It can serve as a road map for us all.

*Onset.* Rapid onset hits hard and shocks everyone, Dr. Rolland states. It demands that the well spouse handle crisis while still in shock. The world comes to a halt and crisis takes over. We see this with Francie, who says:

> Four times in four months, Eric has been in the hospital. He had surgery for a bleeding ulcer. Now he's on dialysis three times a week. They put a plastic tube in his arm, a shunt to make dialysis easier. It got infected. Both his major doctors were off skiing. He developed a roaring infection. It spread to his shunt. Three hours of surgery to save the shunt. He's out of his mind depressed. I've driven four thousand miles back and forth to the hospital across Los Angeles traffic. I've lost eight pounds. I just live all the time with fear.

It's different with slow onset illnesses, Dr. Rolland states. Not much happens right after diagnosis. You row at the same pace, although the farther shore grows oddly unfamiliar and nothing seems quite itself anymore.

*Course.* Some illnesses or conditions do their damage and stabilize. Examples include mild heart attacks, stroke, spinal cord injury with paralysis. The well spouse may exhaust herself or himself at first and then gradually get the practical matters under control. The worst has happened, Dr. Rolland points out. It can never be undone. But at least it's behind you.

Some illnesses come and go in bouts: ulcerative colitis and certain cancers and perhaps two-thirds of the cases of multiple sclerosis. Unpredictable stable periods alternate with unpredictable flare-ups. The family must master two gears: the "well" gear when they act relatively normal and the "sick" gear when options close tight around the illness. Dr. Rolland points to the "taxingly wide psychological discrepancy" between these two gears, a gap the family as well as the patient must learn to straddle. Francie's experience will elucidate that gap.

Some illnesses progress slowly downward, such as emphysema or Parkinson's. You adapt slowly to loss of the sick partner's capability. Decreased mobility? You adapt some more. Decreased energy? You adapt still further. Down, ever downward. Step by step the family takes over the sick person's responsibilities — up to and including the daily care of the physical body. Dr. Rolland notes that the slowest degenerations require enormous stamina from the family: the worst *always* lies ahead. Ted's story and mine elucidates this. For faster-worsening courses, as with certain cancers, the family must adapt more frequently and more massively. This requires enormous flexibility.

*Outcome.* The always-fatal illnesses such as AIDS and metastatic cancer offer no hope. According to Dr. Rolland, the sick fear dying and the well pass into an anticipatory grief that marks every act from diagnosis on. Ambivalence appears as families yearn to be closer yet contradictorally yearn to be able to let go — so the death won't be so painful. What to do when? If the family takes over too much responsibility too soon, Dr. Rolland warns, the sick one becomes emotionally isolated. With the less predictable diseases, the family may tend to overprotect the sick person. The sick one may also become seduced by the secondary gains or benefits of illness — being freed of responsibility, being cared for. The family, as Dr. Rolland suggests, may grow resentful at having to give so much care and take over so much responsibility.

*Incapacitation.* All higher animals must be able to move, sense, produce energy, and integrate these three through cerebral processing. Illness limits in one or more of these areas. When a person can't think for himself, Dr. Rolland reminds us, those who love him become responsible for his every act, night and day. With less disabling illnesses, he notes, the family doesn't quite know when to take over nor what is realistic to expect of the sick. Can she really be *that* tired?

After providing understanding of the particular illness lying ahead, Dr. Rolland in his practice seeks insight into the particular family. What kind is it? Sociologists and psychologists and psychotherapists throw out a variety of labels: functional, dys-functional, adequate, optimal, constricted, internalized, impul-sive, chaotic, skewed — you name it. Observing his clients in hospital rooms and in his office, Dr. Rolland pays particular attention to two factors. He notices how cohesive a family is and how flexible. Sitting forward on a chair in his office, he explains.

Some couples appear to be very cohesive or close. A close family may do well in a crisis, whether it be the opening crisis of diagnosis or the closing crisis of death. They may sit together by a bedside weeping or laughing day and night. They may express their emotions very easily together. Yet sometimes a close family can get too tight, moving and acting as a unit and not allowing others — such as doctors or friends — in. Gener-ally, the closeness or looseness of a husband and wife expands to become the family's dynamic.

Other families appear far less engaged. There's more space between members. A looser family may become too disen-gaged, floating like atoms around the home without really meeting or expressing emotions. This kind of family may experience trouble dealing with the crises of illness but may have more ability to allow each other independence during the long chronic haul.

A family veers toward being flexible or rigid. If flexible, family members adjust well to change and can be quite innovative about family rules and quite practical about solving problems. The flexible family may do very well in the chronic haul. Rigid families may find the long haul harder, especially if they believe in the traditional sexual division of labor and expect certain things to be done in certain ways at certain times. Change comes hard to the rigid family.

These two factors have a lot to do with feeling and acting. Feeling and acting — it's hard to do both during a crisis. Francie describes it: "One thing I've learned is that you've got to have an emotional outlet and you've got to keep feeling. You think all the time, arrange, plan, act. The channels get blocked between thinking and feeling, and pretty soon you're not feeling." Somebody other than Francie might keep on feeling but stop acting. One husband reports: "I can't do a damn thing. I just think about my wife all the time."

How we respond to chronic illness also depends upon our own family history, Dr. Rolland points out. Was a parent sick? A sibling? "You can't look at any family insightfully without an awareness of its history," Dr. Rolland says. "A man who gets sick may have had a father who died from a rapidly progressive form of cancer. From that, he can develop the idea that there isn't anything you can do about sickness." Or a woman, like Francie, may have spent childhood years with a mother who had emphysema and dreads nursing anyone else ever again. Diagnoses fall upon people who have sick-well roles already written into their neurons.

There's another critical element Dr. Rolland considers — when in the life cycle illness hits: "Younger couples in their twenties often struggle more than older couples over whether to break up or to stay together." The diagnosis of a disabling or life-threatening illness shakes the marriage to its foundations because the relationship hasn't really solidified.

"Once you're in the thirties and into child rearing there is another kind of bonding to hold you together, another kind of future," Dr. Rolland continues. "Yet the greatest strain on a couple's energy comes when there are young children to raise. This strain proceeds through the child-rearing years. Raising children is supposed to involve both parents helping equally — however you divide the work. If a severely disabling illness hits during this period, the illness enters the family life like a 'new' member, a parent is lost, and the semblance of a single-parent family with an added child who has 'special needs' is created." For the well spouse, tasks multiply.

"In the postchildren years," Dr. Rolland concludes, "you are supposed to have some leisure, some reaping — vacation, travel, rest, freedom from child rearing. The sense then, I guess, would be that of working very hard and then feeling cheated out of your just rewards."

In discussing the suddenly altered future with his clients, Dr. Rolland looks for signs of what he considers three common problem behaviors: denial, blaming, and isolation. When Leah told her story in a house in Brooklyn over the subway, she appeared entirely free of two of these. If she did deny a bit, this rose quite naturally from the particulars of her family history.

We were twenty-nine when we heard and not yet married. One night Michael was so sick he looked green and I had to hold him in the waiting room because he couldn't sit. When they told us he had diabetes, my first thought was "Oh, that's not so bad!" My father had had open heart surgery and my mother a mild diabetes and an advanced lymphatic cancer. I'd left college and gone back to Colorado and spent five years taking care of them. Toward the end I had some screaming fights with my mother, and they helped because I was able to assure her I would be there while she needed me, but that I had my limits and wanted to live, too. I was twenty-three when she died.

So it took me a while to realize that Michael was upset about the diabetes. It seemed simple to me because he isn't brittle, the way my mother got to be. That means his situation has regularness and it's easy for him to moderate himself. I was so relieved. It meant he'd probably live into his late sixties or maybe into his seventies. Of course I would marry him. We'd been in love for years. It was probably easier, in family terms, for me to bring a sick man home than it would have been for someone else. Michael's family and friends were devastated, but mine figured with diabetes there's so much you can control.

We set a wedding date, and three weeks before it we found out that Michael had a tumor of the thyroid that could be malignant. For him it meant a sense of mortality and vulnerability. It meant "What other secrets are harboring in my body waiting to explode?" For me it meant a funny sense of "Am I always going to be the workhorse? The one who's going to have the right stuff in every crisis? Am I going to have a dependent husband rather than a partner?"

We got into our wedding finery, and a few days after the ceremony we heard the tumor was benign.

Right now, money is our problem and not diabetes. Michael works full-time teaching, and so far he can handle it. I work part-time and would love to quit. I would love to give eight or ten hours a day to my real work. I'm a sculptor. Yet that makes me feel guilty. Michael would like to write, too, but he doesn't have the energy after a day of teaching. Maybe I ought to work full-time. But it would kill me. I'm an artist. I can handle it now, but what about later?

The real pressure will come when it's time to have children. We both long for them, someday. How would I manage working part-time and sculpting and handling almost all the child care? And how could I manage if Michael isn't working full-time and I am? We're each thirty-one and we're not ready for children. We're spending some money now on the therapy we both went into because of the illness. But we mustn't wait too long. Impotence isn't a problem yet, but it might be later on.

Right now, it's only money bothering us — the problem of all young couples.

I guess I can feel so positive about Michael's illness because he has a clear sense of boundaries and responsibilities. I am his friend and lover and wife but not his nurse. He is responsible about his diet. Once when he was low I saw him eating ice cream. That's allowed if you're balancing, but he wasn't. So I asked him if he were feeling depressed and he said he was. Immediately, he took care of his diet again. So, you see, diabetes is just not that important to our lives right now.

Upstairs Michael stands beside Leah in the new kitchen that's just that morning been floored. Their house had been a funeral parlor and that's why it priced out cheap enough to buy. By the new stove, they touch each other often. They smile at each other. The subway passes far below and shakes the books on the shelves in the living room. Michael says that a light bulb left over the couch by the former owners blinks "Closing Hours" every night at 9 P.M. unless he unscrews the bulb.

They laugh.

Everything appeals to their young, zany senses of humor. If any couple can manage chronic illness well, it is this independent, intimate pair.

Yet so much depends upon the course of illness.

# Chapter 3
# Going Public

"So." Ted looked down at me, inside the door. You could see the question in his light eyes. "Daddy!" One of the kids came running behind us.

"You don't look so bad for a man in your condition." I gave him my answer as we hugged for the first time, after. He felt solid to the touch, indestructible. How could it be that he was going to be destroyed? I held on until whichever child it was broke through.

"I do have a balance problem," Ted informed the children as we sat down to supper at the round table in the dining room. He looked exactly as usual, the curly hair receding a bit at the temples, the blue shirt open at the neck — yet our whole lives had changed.

We'd agreed in one of our phone talks that long afternoon to tell the truth to the kids but not the whole truth. What if they saw a TV report on multiple sclerosis? With wheelchairs? We didn't want their lives to change, not yet. Telling would be like opening an umbrella of doom over their heads. Bad luck, opening an umbrella indoors, my mother always said.

"But there isn't much the doctor can do about it," Ted was explaining. "I'll just have to live with it."

Seth pushed his aviator glasses up on his nose. Debbie leaned on an elbow.

I served tuna salad on the Portuguese plates.

"Let me know," Ted instructed, turning to each child the

way he might speak to his staff at the office, "if you've got any questions."

There were none.

He picked up his fork.

Debbie crunched into her lettuce.

Silence. Why silence? Ted and I looked across the table at each other. What were we doing wrong?

"Well, how was day camp, kids?" I finally said. Maybe this wasn't the time, maybe it would come in stages.

"There was a dead squirrel by the fence — " Seth began.

"I put my face under the water!" Debbie bounced in her seat.

It was over, for now.

"Maybe it's all a mistake." Ted sat on the dark couch.

"Maybe." I stood by the fireplace.

But we knew. It explained too much.

"We've got to call. They're waiting." Ted's parents had been sitting by their phones for two weeks. If his knew, mine should know. Ted got up and walked across the living room in bare feet, toward the phone in our bedroom, and shut the door. He walked so well in bare feet. Maybe if he walked an hour a day in bare feet . . . ? I got up and filled my wine glass and walked into the dining room and shut the door.

"There's really nothing to worry about," Ted was saying when I picked up my phone. "I'm fine," he insisted to his parents in Florida. "Hey, it's much, much milder when you get it in your forties." His voice tightened slightly. "There's lots of research going on now," I put in. "There could be a break-through any day now."

"Be well." His parents on their separate phones struggled to control their voices toward the end of what was probably the worst phone call they'd ever gotten in their lives. "The only thing that matters, dear," his mother said, "is . . . your health."

We hung up and met in the kitchen. I got out the maple walnut, Ted's favorite. "It's hard for them," we explained witlessly to each other. "They're awfully upset when, really, it's not all that serious!" We picked up our spoons at the counter. "It probably won't have any effect for years!"

So we managed to calm ourselves enough to dial Boston cheerfully.

"No problem," Ted insisted to his sister Susan and her

husband. "Ted's probably the kind that gets remissions," I instructed at my end. "Two-thirds of the cases do." "It'll probably make very little difference in our lives," Ted informed them of what we wanted to hear. "Not for years."

In Connecticut, it was my mother's first inkling. She started to cry. I'm afraid I told my mother not to be silly. I'm afraid I sounded impatient. "Everything is going to be fine, really! Yes, of course, I'm okay! Yes, of course, Ted will keep working!"

In Minneapolis my brother inquired about life span. "Twenty-five years," I shouted into the phone. "Ted'll be seventy-one. Who wants more than that?"

They all got the message. Four devastating phone calls and we'd made it quite clear: no fussing allowed. It escaped our notice that this had been Dr. Astor's very message to us.

"This isn't so bad." Ted sank into the dark couch again. "I can handle this."

"It's not a brain tumor." I sank down beside him. We held hands, looking into the gas-burning fireplace we'd never dared light a match to.

We felt pretty good: that's what was so strange.


We should call a few friends.

"Stan," Ted said.

"Sid and Mim."

"Agreed." Ted stood up and headed toward the bedroom again. Of course, we agreed. Gone were the domestic squabbles. We moved as a team. I moved back into the dining room and picked up my phone.

"Hang on," Stan was saying. The Mozart that was coming loud over the wire suddenly dimmed. Stan would be our guide from his wheelchair: handsome, amusing, seductive. He would know. "You hear the one," Stan began, "about the baseball player and the rabbi —"

"There's something I've got to tell you," Ted interrupted. He told.

"God." Stan's voice broke. We went right on, rattling off facts, chuckling here and there. MS, which we were already calling by its diminutive, is a degenerative illness, we informed Stan. He kept swallowing, letting us be. It scars or eats away the protective sheath of insulation from the nerves so that your nerves can't tell your muscles what to do. Oh, no, there's no cure. No cure at all. It just progresses in ten downward steps.

You have some trouble walking and sometimes your vision blurs and you get a cane and then two canes and then you can't walk at all and you get a wheelchair and then you can't move much of anything and you lie in bed. You die when your nerves can't make your lung muscles work. Or maybe you get an infection, a complication. But never mind, Stan. Don't worry. Ted is surely on the best track. You know Ted. That's Track B. It means he'll get flare-ups now and then, and then some remissions. Good as new. The casual observer will never know there's anything wrong. Track C? Why, that's steady slow decline, but of course he couldn't have that. Track A? Sudden death, so we know he doesn't have that! What's the matter, Stan?

We could let friends gasp and moan. We needn't shield friends.

"I love you," Stan finally managed to get in, his voice crowded with tears.

In the dining room, I started to undo.

"Sid? Mim?" They answered on separate extensions, their dog barking behind them, their kids shouting. "We've got something to tell you." Ted's voice sounded ebullient.

"Shit," Sid and Mim repeated on their extensions. It's the perfect response. Could they come over?

"Not now." I moved my empty wine glass on the table. "Maybe tomorrow night?"

"Don't tell a soul in publishing," Ted did warn them from the bedroom. "I don't want them to find out at the office."

Mim signed off with what we needed. "At least you know what you'll die of. You've got the jump on the rest of us."

Everything was okay. We weren't the children we'd fallen back to, too far, too fast, when talking with our parents. We were just age mates from the village who had wandered in the woods and been bitten by rattlers.

And gee but we were wonderful!

While Ted watched the late news, I did the dishes and drank more wine. Holy George, who was I kidding? This was horrible. This was more than I cared to accept as my lot in life. I stopped with the dishes. Stan would know what to do. He'd been through it. I dialed him from the kitchen phone. When he answered, I began to sob. I told him the story of the wife who had to be turned over every noon.

"Stop it!" Stan wasted no time. "Stop that right now. Get hold of yourself."

Ashamed, I stopped mid-sob. Stan was the expert on this stuff. I'd been weak. I must be strong. Months later, I realized it would have been far better if I'd cried — but by then I was beyond tears. Years later, I realized that Stan was exactly the wrong person for me to call: he saw himself as Ted, not as me. I must be strong for both of them. That night I made a cup of tea and went to bed.

"Everything will be all right," I said, but I felt as if it were opening night and I was on stage.

"I know." Ted reached for me. "Don't worry."

We slept under the madras spread with our arms around each other. We were both too old to ask Why Me?

Why Hiroshima? Why Nagasaki? Why Auschwitz? Why harelips? Why crossed eyes? Why rheumatic hearts? This here is what you call the darkling plain — ain't nobody here but each other and a couple of friends.

My therapy groupies heard the news before Dr. Miller came home from the waters. "Oh, my," one or two said with unanalytical spontaneity. "Oh, my." Then the familiar note was taken up, the old song. "Of course, you'll leave him now, won't you? Or are you going to stay on and be a martyr?"

"This isn't when you leave someone you love!" I was sitting on a leather stool in somebody's posh den. The room seemed too small; the familiar faces unfamiliar. All of life was taking on a tinge of unreality.

"It isn't? Do you want to wither up and die?"

I stopped talking to them and started talking to myself. This is not what I need. I need support. I need money. There must be a safe way to leave Dr. Miller. Nobody knew how to get out of Dr. Miller's practice. He seemed to suffer from rather severe separation anxiety: he'd been seeing some of his patients for twenty-five years. He'd even started in on people's kids, moving smoothly into the second generation. If you went to Dr. Miller as a couple and one of you quit therapy, the marriage usually ended. So how to get out?

When Dr. Miller returned in September, I'd made up my mind. I gave him one last chance and asked if we couldn't examine the impotence as part of the MS. When he again pooh-poohed this, I went into the very sort of role play he had taught me. I told him how wonderful therapy had been, how good for Ted and me, how much Ted would need it now, how much I'd like to stay but, you see, money was going to be a problem and, therefore, I was leaving. Surprisingly, he confirmed that I was ready to graduate, as he put it — although my timing was bad and I was going to need support. He rose out of his Naugahyde and I out of mine and we gave each other a tiny, guarded hug. Then I walked out, free.

For the first time in years, Park Avenue looked sunny and bright when I left Dr. Miller's office. The defense of myself against a false interpretation and my own capitulation to that interpretation had ended. I was free of that kind of deceit, at least. On 72nd Street, people walked at their vigorous Manhattan clip. There was hope now. I was stronger. I had drawn my energy back into myself. Things would be easier financially and emotionally without this thrice-weekly drain. And there were therapies more ancient than psycho: music, water, travel, friendship, integrity, love. We would do fine.

My years of therapy with Dr. Miller had cut down my contact with old friends, including two women friends who had been in and out of my life twenty years or more. I invited each separately to lunch at the old Library Cafe at 93d and Broadway.

"I've got something to tell you," I told Trisha, with whom I'd shared an apartment after college while we learned to tell the IRT subway from the IND. "Ted has multiple sclerosis."

"Oh, Maggie." Her Welsh eyes filled with tears. "I'm so sorry, so sorry." A bit of the past few weeks' survival euphoria drained away. The numbness I hadn't even known I'd been feeling lifted a millimeter. So it was true. So it was real. So it was awful, just as I'd tried to tell Stan. My husband had multiple sclerosis. How I hated even the sound of the name of it.

Trisha didn't suggest that I take my children and myself away from this stricken man. She knew and loved Ted. It was an enormous relief to be back among people who were simply friends. This particular sorrow was not avoidable. It was not my fault. It was not escapable. It was life.

The next day I told tiny, dark Jane, a rural Iowan with an A average at the university. Trish had brought Jane home from her office once and the three of us had figured out Central Park and which subway cars went to Far Rockaway.

"Oh, Maggie, Maggie. I'm so sorry. And Ted, oh poor Ted." Jane's musical voice sounded elegaic.

Neither of us could eat. We just drank our glasses of wine under the tin roof of the Library Cafe, tin on which the sun shone so autumnally.

"You know, there are some good things in it," I went on, looking out the window at the native New Yorkers in the wonderful city that Trish and Jane and I had adopted together. "Now I see why Ted would never do anything physical around the house. And also, he's always been so future oriented. Never thinking about now. Always about a house in the country. About the next book, the next trip abroad. He's stopped all that. He doesn't fantasize the future anymore. This might be very good for him. Don't you think?"

"Maggie," Jane said, in the voice she must have used for her valedictory, "it's awfully hard to live with someone who's sick. Their faults multiply and grow larger as they get sicker."

Her father, I suddenly recalled, had sat for years in a rocker wearing a button-front sweater and suffering peevishly from an unlockable combination of diabetes and despair.

"Don't worry," I assured her. "That won't happen to Ted!"

She gave me a long, long look and drank off her glass of wine. Finally she said, "How are the kids?"

"Well, they're fine. Fine."

She just looked at me.


It was surreal. We were struck down, yet we prospered. Nothing but the future — which, after all, is only an idea — had changed. How could we grieve when we ate the same and talked the same and did everything we'd done before? Ted was receiving lots of praise for his latest draft of the wartime history of Greece, and we weren't mad at each other anymore. Things seemed great. Debbie held a tag sale of her baby dolls and Seth walked to the Museum of Natural History alone, for the first time.

Labor Day weekend we drove five hours out of the city to visit Ted's sister Susan's weekend place in New England. I drove, but only because Ted was on cortisone and sleepy. He had a cold. Dr. Astor's stand-in had given the pills to him to keep his cold from worsening and doing him any damage. Through Manhattan traffic, northeast over throughways, northwest over dark hills, I drove and we all sang and played word games and yodeled. Seth recounted the adventures of Doctor Doolittle. At midnight we finally arrived at the little house on top of the mountain and fell out of the car, exhausted, making jokes. The kids in their windbreakers and Ted and I in ours, we strode across the floor of Susan and Matt's country house, a four-part dynamo of energy unpent from the car.

"I can't believe you people!" a pale, red-haired Susan whispered, with tears in her eyes. "Here I am an absolute wreck worrying about everything and you all come in like springtime."

It was her first exposure to high denial.

"What's to worry?" we made mockery of her. "So far, everything's fine!"

That night a strange sound woke me from sleep in the guest bed pushed coffinlike into a windowed alcove. Outside dark firs rose to the dark sky. Ted wasn't breathing. Yes, he was. Wasn't he? He took a big rattling breath and then nothing. He didn't breathe out.

I leaned over him to listen. I must have counted to sixty before he let the breath out. How harsh it sounded! He took in another rattling breath and held that.

Was this a death rattle? What should I do? I put my cheek in front of his nose to feel the breath. He was alive. I hung there over him. If he were dying, should I let him? That would save him the terrible decline he faced.

Ted! My Ted, dying?

It must have gone on for half an hour. I didn't know what to do. When you finally become a grown-up, you realize how small and powerless you actually are.

When it ended and his breathing grew normal, I lay back against pillows. Around me moved the total darkness of a country night. I couldn't do this. It was too hard. I couldn't be entirely responsible for someone's living or dying. The only witness, the only decider. It was terrifying. In the morning, I'd tell Susan. It was her responsibility, too. After all, she was a blood relative.

My euphoria was over.

"It's probably just my cold," Ted reasoned when I told not Susan but him as we walked along a fir-lined road to a beaver pond. It turned out that he was right.

Walking back from the pond, I snapped photos of Ted walking. In a still photo, you would never see how he was

favoring his right foot. In his jeans and sandals, with his short curly beard and his wire glasses, he looked pretty much as he had eleven years earlier when we'd driven south on a vacation and conceived a child. Ted Walks: when I snapped the picture, I realized I was recording this fact for a now unknowable future.

So did he.

The sense of the surreal continued. The red-flocked walls of the Chinese restaurant enclosed some hundred diners as we sat with Sid and Mim and Andrew and Grace.

"Gracie! Not in the soup!" Mim extracted the stuffed elephant's trunk from the wonton.

"Let's get the whole black fish," Ted was saying.

"I'm not eating that snake again!" Debbie puffed herself up.

"He hit four ninety-one," Sid was informing Seth and Andrew. "And then he hit. . . ."

Life went on. Nothing changed. But were we really sitting here?

Seth put a new baseball sticker onto his bus pass and started fifth grade. Would he ever get MS? No. No. No. It's not hereditary. I drove to Connecticut to help my mother move from her apartment to a retirement village. Good, she would have people around and not have to depend on me. Debbie liked third grade and won a prize at Hallowe'en for her costume — she went as a head of lettuce after we spent hours stitching together yards of green gauze. Nobody got sick that winter. We were actually happier than we'd been during the awful winter past. And then spring came.

Heads fell at Ted's publishing house. The new management took the company into a more commercial direction, into how-to books that Ted dubbed "How to Spay Your Own Cat" books. In one more year, he would vest his profit sharing and his pension.

"Who wrote 'chocolate cake' on the grocery list?" I stood by the refrigerator and tried to make out the crooked letters. Seth or Debbie?

"I did," Ted called from his desk. "Why do you ask?"

"Oh, nothing."

I'd vowed to be entirely honest. "Promise me," he'd said the day we got the news, "you'll never pull the wool over my eyes." Imperceptibly, I was moving away from sharing all the news with Ted. When you lie next to someone who might be dead or dying, you get stamped with an indelible aloneness.

When we were together, part of me was always watching.

That winter, Ted worked hard to bring the profits of his division up to eleven times its salaries. For years he'd prided himself on walking home from the office. Now it was tiring for him to walk to the subway entrance, to step down the dark stairs, to stand in a crowd and hold onto a strap through six or seven stops to midtown, to walk the several busy blocks to his office. His walk became more and more lopsided. Could they tell? His secretary said nothing. When he got to his desk overlooking Fifth Avenue, he had to sit fast and rest. Then he worked.

And he worried.

His salvation came on Sundays when he revised the final draft of the Greece book. His agent expected it to sell. If Ted didn't have bodily power, he would succeed at writing, at what meant the most to him. In one way, this was the best year of his life.

For me, it wasn't so good. I hadn't landed any full-time jobs — fourteen thousand dollars was my best offer. I was overqualified or underqualified or out of the market raising kids too long. I took on more and more encyclopedia articles, more and more medical editing. I never seemed to get any-where past the middle of things. At one point I found myself in the middle of editing a chapter on mental illness; in the middle of a twenty-page pamphlet on James Joyce's *Dubliners;* in the middle of a four-page article on Alfred Binet and the IQ test; in the middle of negotiations to write a stupid book about people who win lotteries. School would end in a few weeks and I couldn't afford any sitters, yet I had to be free to work. We owed Miller six thousand dollars. I couldn't ask anything more of Ted than he was doing. It seemed as if my brain were shredding into Kleenex.

For relief I started attending a luncheon club of free-lancers that met Wednesdays on Broadway hardly a block away. We exchanged news of work and contacts, although most of the time we laughed over the ongoing mystery we composed at table — about a bald school bus driver who murdered his charges one by one. One day in May, I returned home to a ringing phone.

"Sit down," Ted's managerial voice instructed.

I sat at my desk.

"They gave me the ax." His voice didn't waver. "But don't get upset. I'll get another job."

"Oh, Ted. I'm sorry." Why hadn't I believed him? How could they do this to him, now?

"Don't worry," he repeated. "I'll take care of you. I've spent the last two hours writing résumés. I've set up a lunch date already with someone from Macmillan. I told him I'd meet him at the restaurant. That way I can take the taxi over and he won't see me walking. And then at the end of the lunch I'll tell him I'm staying on to go to the men's room and we won't have to walk out together. He's six four and walks fast."

"Good idea." My eyes rested on the Portuguese plates. It was much easier to deal with this than with a man who wouldn't carry an envelope. My husband was responsible, very responsible. But should he have to go through a job hunt at forty-six? Stumbling into interviews? And then take on the grueling first year in a new job?

"I'm sure you can get a job, Teddie. But why don't we cut out of the city now? We'll go free-lance, just as we've planned, only a little sooner. This could be great. We'll move up to the country and you can write all the time and not have to go on the subway and all."

A silence.

"A man" — his voice sounded slightly less sure — "should support his family."

"A man" — I struggled for words that could release him — "should go after his ideal."

Another silence.

"I don't know." He sounded lighter, happier. "It doesn't seem right. Would you mind?"

"I'd love it."

"Well, we'll see. I'll think about it. Meanwhile, I'm sending out these résumés."

When Ted walked through the door that evening, he looked really beaten. They had given him a good financial package and would pay him at half pay for his tenth year so he could have his profit sharing and his pension. But he'd be out of the office in two weeks, sitting at home.

"I've lost my job," Ted told the children Sunday morning as we sat around in the living room, the piñata swinging over Ted's desk. "But things will be pretty much the same. I'll be able to write more and I'll be around when you get home from school."

"Lost your job?" Seth seemed to be imagining a job as a baseball, as something you hold in your hands.

"The company wants to put out books that I'm not interested in. I'd rather write books, anyway. I'll take care of you."

"What will happen to your office?" Debbie loved to visit there. "To the metal rulers and the glue that goes down with a brush?"

"Somebody else will sit there."

"Somebody else?" She couldn't imagine that.

"You could be an explorer," Seth offered. "Or go on television. You could write about George Washington."

"Yup," Ted said. "I'll go on the 'Today' show and tell them about Greece during World War Two. How about that?"

Did they connect the two bits of news?

Were they connected?


The Monday came that Ted stayed at home instead of going to the office. He did a phenomenal amount of work, so many hours on his revision, so many hours to making contacts for free-lance work. The same the next day. Saturday evening he broke down and cried, when the kids had gone to bed. I found him in the bathroom. He had the shower running so the kids wouldn't hear. He was standing against the glass of the mirror with a towel in his hands. I couldn't cry. I was in charge.

Ted would dream for years and years about being back in his office — in these dreams he is always walking, people surround him, he is taking the subway, he is producing books, men call him for conferences, he takes authors to lunch, he prepares budgets, and he is never tired.

Or fired.

# Chapter 4

# The Acute
# Emotions

The acute emotions amount to love wrapped up in fear and sorrow. A chronic illness may begin with an acute episode — will he live? Will he die? Or the shock of diagnosis may produce the acute emotions. Any acute episode is like a blizzard or a blackout where people pull together. The rest of life sits on hold. Generosity prevails. The acute emotions deliver a high-energy package to see you through crisis. Like acute illnesses, the acute emotions don't last forever. But filled with them, you can do anything. You're alive, aren't you? Alive? You were born on Krypton.

---

## THE ACUTE EMOTIONS

Mostly they bring people together.

DISBELIEF: "You're kidding!" "This can't be happening!"
LOVE: "My darling!"
LOSS: "Where are you?" "Where is the future?"
ANTICIPATORY GRIEF: "He's dying. I'm living. We're each alone."
GUILT: "She's dying. How can I be living?"
ALERT BUT HELPLESS FEAR: "Is he breathing?" "Is she dead now?"

ASSAULT TO TRUST: "Why me?" "What's wrong with God?"
DENIAL: "None of this is real!" "Everything will be all
right."
RESPONSIBILITY: "I alone am responsible."

———◆———

"During traumatic events such as floods and earthquakes,
most persons are able to cope relatively well with the immediate
needs of the community and themselves," according to Dr.
Mardi Horowitz of the Langley Porter Psychiatric Institute at
the University of California at San Francisco. (See Appendix B.)

> There may be an initial period of outcry of emotions, but then
> there is often a dampening down with consideration of some of
> the long range implications of the stressor events. This allows
> survivors to cope with such things as helping the injured,
> digging out the dead, and to keep going to prepare the commu-
> nity to survive in spite of terrible sights and sounds. Very few
> people actually fall into panic, provided that they are not
> rendered helpless in the face of overwhelming calamity. Later,
> after the period of immediate coping with a disaster, there may
> be a continued period of denial and emotional numbing for
> some time, in which implications of the event to the self are
> warded off.

So survivors function very well during the emergency itself.
An acute illness may be short enough to remain an emergency
throughout. The following account provides a glimpse of a well
spouse during eighteen months of his wife's cancer. It differs
notably from later accounts of well spouses five or ten years
into chronic illness.

A poet and teacher at Oberlin College, David Young had
been married to Chloe for twenty years the spring that they got
the news of her breast cancer. Radiation and chemotherapy
followed. The cancer metasticized to the liver and then to the
brain.

> I felt helpless, a tremendous sense of helplessness. As the
> disease became something we lived with, she could put her
> fears aside and go on with life. After the liver scan, we were
> conscious of having only a certain amount of time together. That

sometimes made the times very good, very special. We went to Vermont that summer and lived in a cabin. I was teaching at Breadloaf and she finally read *Ulysses*. We did things we liked.

The children really had no idea about Chloe's timetable. She just couldn't tell them. She couldn't not protect them. That fall our son went off to Vassar. I had a teaching assignment in London and we returned for a semester to a city where we'd lived before and which she loved. We were proud of ourselves for not letting the disease make her homebound.

When we came home in January of '84, she continued chemo. The percentages they give you, they sort of shrink. In the middle of a night during that next summer, she had her first seizure. She was in bed having convulsions, she was unconscious. I was tremendously frightened. I thought she might have had a stroke.

Radiation for that.

Our daughter started school at Yale and really liked it. How well the children had turned out made the last months of Chloe's life happy.

That Christmas was somehow very special. Everybody knew she was dwindling.

All through the illness I was grieving.

My great dread was that I would have trouble nursing her toward the end. Would I feel helpless? I'm not a nurse. Did I want to witness the pain? Could I? Without being able to alleviate it?

In the course of a blood transfusion after Christmas, Chloe had heart failure. They put her on a respirator. She never came out of her unconsciousness. After a few days, we took an EEG and realized there'd been massive brain damage. We decided to unplug the respirator. I had assembled the family and everyone was ready for that.

But then the person is gone and you realize that no amount of preparation can be sufficient.

The first months I got through day to day in some very strange numb way, like an automaton. In the summer, the children and I took a trip together to South America, rather extravagant. We did it to be together. That was something we thought she would have liked. Somehow all of us came back from that a little bit more reconciled to her death. My main emotion through the twenty months was . . . love. The illness brought our love into high relief.

\* \* \*

If the patient lives, the love-centered acute emotions that David Young describes begin to dissolve under two conditions. The first is when the patient starts to get better. The emergency ends. You can let down your guard. You don't have to be ready to suction your wife if she chokes. Or to catch your husband if he blacks out. You don't, however, return directly to normal. The bettering phase usually brings conflict. You've been holding a lot back, and now you may get angry or depressed. Let's look at what happened when eight men began to get better from their heart attacks.

During the mid-1970s, Edward J. Speedling watched eight men who had suffered heart attacks and their wives as they moved from the crisis phase of the intensive care unit into the general wards of their hospitals and then back home for recovery. Out of his observations Speedling wrote a Ph.D. dissertation, which he turned into a book, *Heart Attack: The Family Response at Home and in the Hospital* (see Appendix B).

In a small windowed office high in the Annenburg Tower at Mount Sinai Medical Center in New York where he now serves as director of organizational development in the Department of Human Resources and as assistant professor in the Department of Community Medicine, Dr. Speedling recalls what he found in those eight normal, emotionally sound families. According to Dr. Speedling, the men became passive in the intensive care units. They accepted a child's role of freedom from responsibility and relied completely upon the doctors and nurses. The men became the center of activity for a proficient staff and the focus of lots of energy and machines. The patients generally knew what was going to happen next and they seemed optimistic and made jokes.

In contrast, their families were left in the dark, or, in actuality, outside the units in poorly furnished waiting rooms with little access to doctors or nurses. One wife that Dr. Speedling tells of in his book sat in a chair located outside a closet where nurses brought a steady parade of stainless steel pots full of feces or urine or vomit to empty. Another sat in a high-tech unit near the open door to a closet. Inside, a box marked "shrouds" could be seen. The wives grew pessimistic and fearful.

The ICUs acquired a halo effect. Both husbands and wives felt frightened in the general wards afterward and unprepared about going home. Once home, they quickly re-created the atmosphere of the ICU. The husband remained passive. The wife took charge. During what Dr. Speedling calls Phase One at home, which usually lasted six to eight weeks, the husbands stayed where the wives could see them — in bedrooms or living rooms. Death might come at any time. "If I drop a piece of paper," one husband told Dr. Speedling, "she won't let me pick it up." Family fighting ceased, even kids stopped fighting. There was joy, sorrow, and fear. Nobody blamed anybody for anything. Crises were thought of as coming from the outside. Rigid families did well in this phase. Cohesive families did better than the less engaged.

In what Dr. Speedling calls Phase Two at home, the men began to feel a little better. They started to push themselves lest they become permanently disabled. And they grew unpredictably angry. They wanted to be in charge of things again. They moved into distant dens or furnished basements. The wives got frightened and angry and punished their husbands for doing too much. The potential for crisis moved to the inside of the family. Fights erupted; friction abounded. One wife actually died — she had a heart attack of her own. Another suffered a nervous breakdown and was institutionalized. Flexible and less engaged families did better in this phase than rigid and cohesive families.

"With heart patients," Dr. Speedling remarks as the late-afternoon sun lights up his desk, "the patient needs to make choices. If he's unwilling to make choices, there is little the spouse can do except fight with him."

The second condition under which the love-centered emotions dissolve is with the shift into long-term illness. You leave the acute emotions behind — although they're never entirely gone. They resurface at any crisis. If the illness is mild, you may not move very far from them. If it's more severe, you may look back from a great distance with yearning: sad as they are, those acute emotions can look mighty good. With chronic illness, you're in danger of moving toward a lifetime of the more divisive atmosphere of Dr. Speedling's Phase Two.

# TO TELL OR NOT TO TELL?

If you tell, folks gather round with love and cookies, and you'll need all of that you can get. But once the word is out, people will look at you differently and you'll feel different, too.

"Kidney failure," "heart attack," "leukemia," "diabetes" — these words will strike the ears of friends or strangers just as they did yours. They will alter the images produced by other words, such as "independent adult" or "energetic worker." And each time we go public, we absorb the shock of diagnosis over again as we watch the question of competency appear on our listeners' faces. As one woman put it: "If I ever get sick, I'm not telling a soul. I saw what happened to my husband after his heart attack."

Yet we need to tell. We need the rallying round. Not to tell is to engage in a massive public denial that may ultimately isolate you more by deception than you would have isolated yourself by revelation. Are there any surprises when you tell?

Yup.

*Telling family.* You assume parents will take on a sorrow from which there's no reprieve, and they do. You may not expect that this may make you feel rather like you did the semester you flunked chemistry or the night they caught you smoking.

You assume your siblings will feel sad. You may not expect that they might also feel guilty that they're well and then perhaps angry — because they've been cornered into feeling guilty. Somehow they've won the ancient sibling war that they weren't even fighting anymore. You've lost, you're weak; they're strong — they have to let you win at Monopoly now.

*Telling children.* This is the hardest. Children have so much future to be altered. They have so much world to figure out. They need so much. Telling them dents the beneficence of the world. It makes them think they can't ask for much from you. With rapid onset, you must tell immediately. With slow onset, you might buy them some time. But do they already suspect something is wrong?

You can't win. Not telling children makes a wall between you. Telling them makes a wall of time in your house: before and after the news.

*Telling employers.* As soon as employers know, your spouse's job may be in danger. Forced retirement may be a second blow to someone who has recently learned he's chronically ill. Such loss can hasten a downward spiral of emotional and financial depression.

It's extremely difficult to find out if someone has been fired because of sickness. The law protects the disabled in certain federally funded jobs — with contractors, hospitals, museums, universities. The Rehabilitation Act of 1973 helps the handicapped find and keep jobs. Facilities must be accessible to the handicapped and equal opportunities for advancement and benefits offered. To find out if a certain organization is so protected, call the Office of Federal Contract Compliance Programs (see Appendix A) or your governor's office. A chronically ill worker, however, may be too fatigued to complete a day's labor.

*Telling friends and others.* You assume they will grieve with you, but you may not expect to feel demoted to vulnerability. People may fuse you with your spouse and you may begin to take on his or her physical vulnerability in others' eyes.

"Shall I carry that for you?"

"I'll bring over the food, you've got enough to manage."

It's wonderful, but no wonder the giver of bad news often ends up comforting his listeners and insisting nothing is really wrong. We do it partly in order to retain our own sense of adulthood.

You may also be surprised at how fast you leave the mainstream. You'll no longer identify with healthy peers who continue to examine each other anxiously for such harmless stuff as gray in the beard. This happens whether you tell or not, but if you tell, the process may speed up.

Do tell someone, even if your spouse doesn't want to. You need the support.

---

# IF YOUR SPOUSE LOSES A JOB

Act fast. If he's well enough to make decisions, see that your spouse considers the following two steps.

Transfer desired group health insurance policies to individual status. If a worker doesn't take these options when he or she leaves a job, they're gone forever.

Investigate Medicare disability insurance. Does your spouse qualify for Social Security disability? Has he or she completed enough quarters of work? Was he working until he couldn't? Will she earn less than several hundred dollars a month from occasional labor? Do you yourself qualify? If he qualifies and you have children under sixteen, you may qualify too. To find out more, call your local Social Security Administration. Look in the white pages for the United States Government listing, and within that, under the Health and Human Services Department. For such calls, be prepared to wait, and when you finally reach someone, record that person's name and ask for the same person next time you call.

# Chapter 5

# I Can Do It!
# I Can Do It!
# (But Do I Exist?)....

Nobody offered Ted a job; nobody offered me one. The kids could go to public school. We could limit all amusement to the wonderful free events of Metropolis. But the elementary school near us fell two grades below national in reading. Better to live a downwardly mobile life in the great American townscape.

"When shall we tell them?" I stood by the gauze curtains in our bedroom.

"When's the school money due?" Ted bent to turn off the TV.

"Monday. I got an extension."

We weren't going to connect the move to the illness.

In the living room, Seth was lying on the dark couch reading *Huckleberry Finn*, his long legs dangling over the edge. Usually, when he did that, he would laugh out loud. Debbie came running from her room dragging a broom she'd dressed up into a dancing partner.

"We want to tell you something." The white paint of the room glowed around us. "You remember how I lost my job?" Ted leaned against his desk in shorts and sandals. "Well, we've decided to move out of the city. It's very expensive here and we can live for half as much in the country. We've got to act fast so you can start school in September when the other kids do."

"What do you mean?" Seth looked up from his book.

"I mean we are thinking of moving to the country."

"I don't want to."

"Why not?"

"This is where we live."

"I want to!" Debbie held the broom close. "I hate Sharon."

"Maybe we'll get a dog," I put in.

"I only want a cat." Seth knew he couldn't have one.

"You know I'm allergic. A nice short-haired dog."

"I'm not sure." Seth looked back at his book. "I'm right at the end of a chapter."

"I want a dog like Lassie!" Debbie's eyes were large behind her lenses. What sweet kids. What happened to men and women in their twenties who got MS? Who never get married? Never had children? We were lucky, lucky.

"I can't believe I won't be coming back here in September," Seth said as we stood in the school lobby waiting for Debbie. Familiar children celebrating summer's liberation ran past us down the steps and off toward Central Park.

"Me neither." Was Seth, too, suffering from the surreal?

Pam, Charlie, Nicole, Jennie, Simeon, Freddie . . . how would they grow up? Who would be tall? Who short? Who fat? Who thin? Who sweet? Who bullyish? Not to know them as they grew? What were we doing to the children? But our lives no longer circled around their needs.

Item 1: No more attempts to make Ted take over traditional female chores — no more haggling over dishes after a dinner party. Those jobs were mine and I'd do them cheerfully (at last). Item 2: No more attempts to get Ted to do traditional male chores he rejected — of course the air conditioner was too heavy for him! I'd take over whatever was too hard. I'd always preferred men's chores, anyway. Item 3: Accomplish same with seamless grace and thus make life easier for Ted, and so subtly he'll never notice.

"I've got it," I said one day at the dishwasher. "I'll do the physical work and you do the mental." Smoke and mirrors: female wiles, as my grandmothers would have put it.

Taking over the driving! That I especially loved. Who wants to sit in the passenger seat holding used apple cores and trying to think up word games? Hey, this was the life. I was upgraded. Must be careful not to intrude on Ted, though. He worried about controlling his right foot on the pedals, but must be careful to take over only what he wants me to. Mustn't demasculinize him. Mustn't infantilize him.

"Is this where we turn?" I would ask Ted whenever I drove. My grandmothers had nothing on me. We drove a lot, looking for a town, a house.

"Don't be surprised to find Ted home," I warned Mel and Doris in the honking smog of West End Avenue. They stood in their Florida tans, not expecting to see their son until the end of the work day.

"He's not feeling sick, is he?" Doris picked up her overnight case and a shopping bag, struggling to look cheerful.

"No, no, he's fine."

Mel carried both suitcases into the elevator, and I took the other two shopping bags, loaded with gifts.

"So why is he home? What's wrong?" Mel moved away from the clanging elevator cage.

"He's gone to the corner for the *Times*." I couldn't stall them any longer. "He's . . . lost his job. . . ." I told them the story as we moved along the neon-lit corridor to the apartment door. "We're moving out of the city. Just think, the kids' lungs won't coat over with exhaust. And we can live on twenty-five or thirty thousand." I opened the door into the foyer.

"But my son . . ." Mel set the heavy suitcases down in the foyer. "I want my son" — he straightened up, perplexed — "to make . . . sixty or seventy thousand."

At first I thought this a strange remark. Didn't he know how sick Ted was? That stress — finding a new job and doing splashingly well at it — wouldn't help? Then I looked closer at Mel's face. What a wonderful face Mel had. He'd emigrated to America as a boy. In the golden land, he'd found a job unloading meat from trucks. Then he'd learned to cut and package meat. He worked up to be a meat manager and buyer. He sent his son to Harvard. He bought a used Cadillac. He retired to Florida. His was the first generation — the generation that labors to transplant the tree, that waits for its children to "take" and flourish, that survives hard times soberly so there will be a future. And now, where was it, that future?

Mel's face expressed supreme confusion. Ted's professional job, gone? He, Mel, wasn't just the conduit anymore? He, Mel, may have been the flowering? the bloom? When the future changes, so does the past. Mel's whole life was taking a new shape inside his head.

"It's not right." He looked back and forth from me to Doris. "He should find a new job."

"Stress is bad for him, Dad. But here he is now. Let him tell you himself."

Sometimes the new future would open up before us, too, and take our breath away.

Luckily, we'd spent vacation days here and there driving through New England towns imagining ourselves ensconced in old Victorians. We knew we wanted rural Massachusetts, and when Susan mailed us information about school systems, we drove up to take a look at the options and settled easily on Highfield. It had good libraries, good schools, and lots of displaced New Yorkers. Driving its shaded streets that July night, we congratulated ourselves: we'd found our town and had six whole weeks in which to find our house.

"*Mall, mall,*" Ted sang in imitation of Petula Clark singing "Downtown" as we passed a dark sprawl of mall on our way back to the city. I turned off and we went in.

"Our first mall!"

"*Mall, mall, life could be better here.*" We chanted improvised words in the artificially lighted corridors where teenagers walked with their arms around each other and babies reached to tired grandparents. Here it was, the new town life, and we were going to be part of it; we were still in the mainstream.

"I'm tired." Ted headed back to the dark parking lot. As I got into the driver's seat, Ted made an anguished noise and fell into the passenger's seat.

"What is it?"

"Wet my pants." He slumped against the seat and covered his face with his hands. "Too fast." His voice broke. "It's all happening too fast."

"I'm sorry. I'm sorry." The future was too awful, and I began to apologize for it.

Ted learned to regulate his liquid intake, and we realized not every symptom would be global or permanent. All that hot summer, I packed. First, Seth's trunk for sleepaway camp.

"I'll drive." Ted hurried along Riverside Drive to the car. "I want him to see me driving."

How scared Seth looked, a light-eyed, curly-haired kid standing at the airport, coolly letting the other kids make their contacts while he took their measure.

"Goodbye, sweetie pie." I held him to me to feel him close before his first big trip. "When we find a house, I'll send you a picture."

He moved away and gave a small desperate smile.

"See you later, alligator," I called after him.

"After a while, alligator!" It was our joke.

We lost sight of him in the long line of well-to-do New York kids.

"I'm just as glad they're getting out of this crowd." Ted led the way to the parking lot. "You drive home."

Back in the closets I kept on sorting, packing. Should we keep Debbie's bright paintings of sunrise over the ocean? Seth's careful pencil cartoons of basketball players drawn from above the court? I packed it all. This was our life I was putting away! I mustn't think of it as "better days." Surely there would be wonderful days ahead?

One house in Highfield had a yard too steep for Ted. Another required more plastering and painting than we could now do. The rest were too expensive. Hot and discouraged at noon one August weekday, we rented a small ranch-style apartment in a condominium complex in the right school district. Coming out of the rental office, I felt dizzy and asked Ted to drive.

He drove. Across the yellow line and into the wrong lane against oncoming traffic.

One thing was clear: I mustn't get sick.

Ever.

"You can't drive a truck!" my brother said from Minneapolis.

"It's only as big as a telephone truck."

"Please don't drive a truck!" my mother pleaded from Connecticut. "A man should do that."

"Let me drive that truck up," my friend Jane urged; she'd been divorced for a couple of years and was used to doing everything. "You're doing too much!"

"Stop it!" I shouted at all of them.

Couldn't they see that everything was fine?

In my jeans and sandals and India cotton shirt and looking

not a day over my forty-four years, I pulled the truck into my mother's driveway in fine style. There she stood in her mid-seventies, a sweater over her shoulders on the pebbly drive. And there, coming out of her apartment, was my brother, gray-haired and jovial.

How could they do this to me?

"I'm so glad he flew in! I'm so glad you don't have to drive that truck!" My mother took us inside and served us lunch.

How about the ninety miles I just managed pretty neatly over the highway, Dad? I addressed myself to the photograph of my father on the piano. He believed in women doing things; he believed in me. You win some, you lose some, he said from the piano.

"Come on, I'll load up the bikes." My brother wouldn't let me lift a finger: there's men's work and there's women's work.

"Let's have the keys," my brother said, holding out his hand.

I slid into the passenger seat by the potted plants. As the hazy summer farmland slid past, I tried to figure out why nobody could say the right thing to me. Because it was impossible. Because I wanted to prove that I could easily make up for the tiny, manageable flaw in the structure of our lives. So nobody, not even me, would notice. Therefore no one must comment on my acts as extraordinary. Yet I was working damn hard and did crave some notice, although not within Ted's hearing. Yet whenever notice or help was offered, I slapped the hand that gave, because it meant that things were not the same.

"Let me know what's in the right lane now."

"Sure thing, boss."

There was the other thing: I'd come to enjoy being in charge.

Then it was time to say goodbye to the city in which both Ted and I had found refuge from New England's narrower expectations for us. Jane gave us a farewell party in her brownstone near Central Park West with beautiful plates of cold chicken edged with watercress. Sid and Mim gave us a farewell party overlooking the Hudson with "I luv New York" tee shirts for the kids.

A hundred people hugged us and kissed us. The reason for all this festivity seemed silly and inconsequential. Surely this was not the end of friendship with people we had loved from twenty to forty? Surely we would be growing gray along with Stan, whose hair was already turning? Along with Jane and Trisha and Sid and Mim and all the others, central and peripheral to our lives? How could we not? How could we stand that?

Easy. Because we could do anything. This was just a play and we were acting in it. Nothing really happened anymore.

On the last Sunday in August, Ted waited in the cool fern-filled lobby out of the sun so damaging to sclerotics. The kids and I and Jane and her son Patrick packed the old Buick that Mel and Doris had given us.

"I remember this from Twenty-third Street!" Jane held up a framed poster from *My Fair Lady*.

The loose items welled up over the backseat and left only two small perches for Seth and Debbie. Ted made the gauntlet sheepishly to the car.

"You did a great job supervising," I assured him as he settled in the passenger seat.

Jane and I hugged goodbye. Seth and Patrick joined hands, the one inside and other outside the car. I pulled slowly away from the curb, tearing their fingers apart. I waved to tiny Jane.

"Jane's crying," I reported to Ted, genuinely surprised. I had no emotions at all anymore. My face had frozen into a no-see, no-feel mask.

The next day I drove the kids over green countryside to the ranch-style school.

"It's not bad," Seth admitted, an agile fellow at the top of a jungle gym against the coloring-book blue sky. Culture is universal: all jungle gyms are the same.

I wondered. A skinny kid? With glasses and flawless grammar? From New York?

"Will the girls wear dresses or jeans?" Debbie pulled worriedly at her shorts and stood closer to me.

We went to the library for cards and to the YMCA for memberships. After Manhattan, everything seemed so cheap and easy. No long lines, no waits at the P.O. Those few days before school were like Sundays, with the three of us exploring while Ted worked at his desk, only now his desk sat on a shag rug and looked out onto woods.

His fingers got tired after an hour or two pounding his manual typewriter. He solved that: "I think I'll work seven days a week." With MS you can't build yourself up by running around the reservoir. You can't even tell whether you're pushing yourself too hard or pampering yourself.

"MS is un-American," Ted decreed. He made himself a grilled cheese in the apartment's galley kitchen, wearing a thick glove to protect his hand from the heat. "Do you think I can walk two miles into town?"

"Does it make you tired?"

"I'm always tired. I wake up in the morning tired."

The foursome changed subtly. We began to meet the people I called, to visit the places I found on the map, to do the things I planned. Ted's energy shrank, and he gave second place to his zest for exploring unknown roads and antique stores and nineteenth-century mill towns. His work took first place and became his definition: nothing must take that away.

And, of course, he did no physical labor.

When I brought eight heavy bags of groceries up the two flights, he stirred guiltily at his desk.

"I wish I could help." He looked tanned and relaxed.

"No problem." Not for the resourceful. Buy a grocery wagon. Be sure to wheel it into the apartment when he isn't looking.

"I wish I could help you wheel that thing up the stairs."

"No problem! Save it for your remission, kid!"

Secret messages ran from ear to ear inside my head like small abbreviated bullets: *Reduced. Terribly reduced.* And *tired. Tired.*

I gave small dinners every Wednesday night so we could get to know those twenty people whose names had been pressed into our hands in New York. We introduced ourselves as writers moved out of the city. We weren't telling anybody in Highfield about the MS until next summer. By then the two years would be up on our disability insurance. Besides, we wanted to appear normal.

Many of them were writers moved out of New York, too. The men helped their wives off with their sweaters. The wives had taught courses and raised sheep and attended consciousness-raising groups and taught kids to do macramé; the men had mastered Akido and gone rabbit hunting and built houses and winched cars out of ditches. Everybody remembered Zabar's on the Upper West Side. How exuberant they were! How fast they moved! How loud they talked! They were healthy!

Ladling up chili from the galley, I listened to their voices coming to me over the shag rug — excited, sociable voices. I stood there listening, unwilling to join in. Their voices brought back something I could remember: happiness.

"There'll be nobody out there but Republicans with haircuts." Ted pulled on his denim cap, touched his beard, adjusted his wire-framed glasses, and headed off to try the walk to town. As slow to warm up as Seth, he began to like Highfield.

"Guess what?" He came through the door a couple of hours later. "Everybody else out there has a beard and the same glasses!" But he was tired.

He took a bus to New York and found more and more free-lance work. Mine was running alarmingly dry.

He joined the Historical Commission. "Couldn't join anything like that in Manhattan," he told a dinner guest. "All unionized."

He sat with us afternoons on a bench in a field shaded by yellowing maples. Out there in green socks and uniform ran our son at soccer.

"If you weren't sick, you wouldn't be able to do this." I unscrewed the top of the coffee thermos and its wonderful aroma steamed up.

"Secondary benefits," he whispered. "Don't say I don't do anything for you."

"Is this a city or a town?" Seth hung over the backseat of the Buick as we drove to buy a quart of mint chocolate chip. I brought a lot of junk food and sweets those first months of the move.

"A town." We passed cows, joggers.

"I like a town." Where had Seth learned that you don't sit in front with your mother? You sit in back with your chauffeur? "A town and mint chocolate chip. I like it here."

"Me, too." And I did.

Ted turned forty-seven and I asked each child to write him a story for his birthday, as a special treat. That's when we found out what was happening. In both their stories the mother did everything and the father sat passively by.

"I'll try to do more," Ted pledged, as we lay under our madras spread in the small room with the high windows.

"I'll try to do less."
But what?

A Realtor called with a white Victorian in the wrong school district a half mile from town. Beautiful maple-arched street, orange and yellow leaves on every lawn, lovely old houses — the very street I'd fled as an adolescent: on such streets intellectual girls refuse to practice the piano and go mad in attics.

"Pretty." I got out of the car. "Very pretty." A sun-filled Victorian, with a long living room containing five windows. A door opened onto a screened porch and there was a small dining room with paneling. Behind it, a big old kitchen with ugly linoleum and ancient fixtures and four beautiful windows, two made cozy by fir trees.

"Of course you'd have to redo the kitchen," the Realtor said.

On the refrigerator someone had taped the photograph of two smiling boys, handsome, grown. On the porch a young-faced, white-haired woman told us her husband had died young and that now the boys were raised, she didn't need the space. She sat on a wicker couch, looking composed, serene. If she could do it, I could.

"Let's take it," Ted said softly in the hall. "I'll be able to walk to town from here."

"Let's."

Fifty-eight thousand at nine and a half, a beauty of a buy. We could move in at Thanksgiving.

"I'm going to be a house," Seth informed us at Hallowe'en. He found a big packing box to wear.

"It was good being a lettuce." Debbie fell back on the past and we reproduced her old costume.

The sky darkened and the jack-o'-lanterns glowed, and we drove to the house so the kids could do their trick-or-treating in their own neighborhood. Lights burned on all the porches down the street. I pulled up not too near the new house. We all got out, except Ted. Then we just stood there.

Seth stepped out of his box. "I want to go home," he said sadly.

Where did he mean?

"I want to go home to my real house." Debbie explained it. "I want to go home to New York!"

Ted opened his door. "Tell you what," he said in a comforting tone, "let's go out for hot chocolate instead."

"We should talk about how we feel."

"I can't." Ted's voice sounded distant although we lay touching in the double bed under the high windows. "It's too big. If I open the door, I'll be destroyed."

"I know what you mean."

Living with the illness felt like the summer during college that I'd worked at a camp for crippled children. The first day I couldn't eat supper. I told my parents about the blind girl and the deaf girl and the boy with the brain tumor and the girl with cerebral palsy and how sad it was. By the third day I was eating fine and applauding when the kid with no arms learned to swim. It all comes down to small successes; you work at it.

"Okay, so let's not talk about it."

"There's one thing." Ted's voice grew colder, frightened. "What?"

"It was dumb to take that house. I'm kidding myself. In two years I won't be able to walk to town from there."

"So we're in the wrong district for nothing!"

Dr. Miller had been right about one thing: trouble makes Ted frightened and Maggie angry. A terrible anger was growing in me.

"I'll help with that." Ted watched me stack boxes of books, preparing for the next move.

"Do you think you should?"

"Who knows?" He looked so healthy.

"Better not, then."

Ted left more and more to me, but in such small units I'd acquiesced before I could object. Then it was too late. And who can get angry at somebody who can't lift a dictionary?

Two days before Thanksgiving, I drove several hours south to Mim and Sid's duplex for the second move. There was my life — the skyline from the Henry Hudson Parkway, the dark towers in November's black and white light, a sense of excitement and power, promise, hope, liberation. New York is a woman's city. "And do you write, too, Mrs. Greenstein?" a number of people in Highfield inquired.

"How's it going, babe?" Brown-eyed Sid kissed me at the

door from which echoed barking dog and laughing/crying kids and Mim shouting into the phone. Everything was normal. Everything was fine. Except I didn't belong here anymore.

"He's frightened," I said after supper.

"Of course he's frightened!" they said. "Wouldn't you be?"

"Yeah, I would be."

I couldn't tell them I was angry that their friend couldn't lift a dictionary.

The next day a meter cop ticketed me and the movers arrived late and the landlord evicted us for subletting. Outside the high windows where the piñata no longer swung, it grew colder and darker as I helped the movers pack all the rest of our furniture. The parquet floor became barer and barer as they carried out Seth's bunk and the dark couch and the round oak table. At 8 P.M. I got in the car and drove north with the long framed Chinese fabric and the other fragiles. Wind blew at the car all the way up.

"How was it?" Ted sat up in bed.

"Hard." Usually I tried to give Ted full, colorful reports, so he would feel he'd been there.

"Snow for Thanksgiving!" The movers propped open the door of the house and brought the couch through languid thick snowflakes. "That's some winter they've got up here."

"It's lovely, dear." My mother arrived around noon. "Lovely." It was clear she might have preferred a small carpeted ranch.

"A wonderful house!" Our friends Tim and Eileen called from their car. We'd had Thanksgiving with them for several years, ever since Ted had given Tim his first job. Eileen hugged me and handed me a woven wheat sheaf for good luck.

"Hi, boss!" Tim embraced Ted on the porch and went to the car for his toolbox.

"Where's Debbie?" Their five-year-old, Maud, considered Debbie the best baby-sitter in the world.

We worked together all day, settling in, all but Ted. My seventy-five-year-old mother had more strength and energy than my husband.

"When I move this spring," my mother said, "I'll send you my piano." She was leaving her retirement community for an apartment in a continuing care community — she knew now that she could not rely on me for much of anything but holidays and occasional visits.

She bent to lift a box of books.

"I'll get that!"

"I can do it, dear." It seemed so unnatural.

Eileen arranged the pantry in her peaceful way. Tim hammered up bookcases and tightened doorknobs. I unpacked books.

"I'm not doing anything." Ted sat in a chair.

"Where do you want this bookcase?" Tim asked tactfully, making himself Ted's arms and hands.

"Let's you and I go downtown for some candy." My mother invited Ted out of it. They walked to a store a quarter of a mile away and Ted had to stop to rest, pretending to admire snow on the branches of a fir.

Seth chose the bedroom nearest ours, smaller and darker, perhaps safer. It was painted an ugly orange. Debbie got the big bright room, this time, with a picture view of the turn-of-the-century architecture: she set up her dollhouse and put her boy doll in one bedroom and her girl doll in another — their parents got the attic. The three kids carried cardboard boxes outdoors and down to the end of the street, where it turned to a dirt road that ran downhill under trees to a meadow, and went sliding.

"The kids look terrific," Eileen said. "As if they'd taken off those nerve overcoats you wear in the city."

Tim and Eileen and Maud slept at our house that first night, to warm it for us.

Thanksgiving morning my mother and I put the turkey into the oven at the apartment, and then we loaded the car to start the third move.

"Try not to carry anything heavy past Ted," I urged her. What an odd switch!

We took a load over and came back for the turkey. We finished baking the turkey in the oven at the new house. We set the table for eleven.

"What a wonderful house!" Susan and Matt and one of Susan's sons arrived.

What energy they brought into the house!

"Better carve it in the kitchen," I suggested to Matt. "So Ted won't feel funny."

At the table, Tim read Stephen Vincent Benét's "American Names," as he always does. I got tears in my eyes, as I always do. Snow lay on the bushes and on the branches of the maple trees outside the curtainless windows. New flakes fell past the hundred-year-old glass. The children laughed and ate too much and kept running up to make sure their rooms were still there.

When our guests all left, we were alone again.

"Shut the kitchen door, will you?" Ted's knees were sensitive to the heat of the oven. He'd feel rings banding them. Or a tingling inside them. Sometimes he'd tell me to shut the kitchen door when the stove wasn't even on.

"Let me run a test," I called back once. "Have I got a burner on or not?"

"Damn it, just believe me!"

We kept the thermostat at sixty-four degrees.

"Can't we put it up, dear?" my mother asked the next time she visited.

"Ted's doctor says heat damage might be irreversible. I'll put it at sixty-eight, but after that Ted feels the rings."

"Old people get cold, dear."

Everything wheeled and circled around Ted's needs. We all began to lose the habit of our own desires.

In our chilly bedroom upstairs with the two tall windows that started low to the floor, there was space for only one night table.

Ted's.

The bureau had a sticky drawer and an easy drawer.

Ted's.

The warm side of the bed was nearer to the door.

Ted's.

At least you could see the trees out the curtainless windows. And in my dreams I was not an automaton.

There was a grubby room behind the kitchen for one study and a beautiful upstairs sunroom for another, Ted's. Eleven windows in that room: I would make storms for him in my carpentry class.

"This is the life." Ted sat up in the sunroom with the formal desk and the Beduin rug.

How could I get mad? He was sick. I was well. I set up my file cabinets behind the kitchen, the easier to throw in a wash now and then.

"How's it going?" Jane asked over the phone.

"Pretty good." I was ashamed to complain to her. "He can't do much."

"Does he do less than he could?"

Jane and Trisha, too, tended to jump in too fast to support me against Ted.

"Of course he doesn't!" I rushed in to defend him.

There was no one I could talk to. My own pain was pain, but there was no one I could tell it to. To Ted's family, it would sound like treason. To my own, it brought upset. Old friends were too close to give the sorrow to. Ted didn't want them to know everything, anyway. Jane got upset for me. Sid and Mim got upset for Ted. So I stopped talking.

Horrible brown, pink, yellow, green, and white wallpaper ran around our bedroom, making it smaller, more like a prison.

Lying by my window under my mother's bedspread dyed brown, I planned a housewarming. We'd have the tiny older woman who'd been hoeing in the garden of one house we looked at. And the professor couple. And the news reporter. And the banker couple who'd brought us bird feeders. And the old couple down the street who'd taught dancing during the depression. And the real estate agent. And the children's book writer and the. . . .

"Guess what?"

"What?"

"I couldn't get my right leg up the porch step today. I had to lift it with my hands."

"I'm sorry. Tell me."

"I don't want to talk about it."

"Tomorrow you get your remission."

He hadn't had one. Or had he? The books were fuzzy. Some made you think a remission meant return to normal, others made it sound like a plateau.

"It's good he's decided not to come on as a smart kid from New York," Seth's sixth-grade teacher confided on Parents' Night. "That shows you just how smart he is."

"She doesn't talk much but she's a flyer in reading," Debbie's teacher said. "Try to keep her in this school next year. It's the best."

They could stay in the school so long as I drove them. In the morning, exhaust blackened the snow as I scraped.

"This is how you scrape it." I demonstrated to Seth and to Debbie — impartial about the sexuality of windshields. Neither one was too interested.

"This is how you vacuum."

"Mom! Why don't we get a housekeeper like we used to have?"

Our four tickets to *Annie* arrived just before Christmas. Ted couldn't go. The fingers of his right hand were tingling and he was on a new kind of cortisone. How he responded would show whether he was, indeed, on Track B. If not, he might be on Track C, steady decline.

"What's that?" I asked Debbie as we drove. She sat in her puffy blue parka with her security blanket bunched fat on her lap.

"My doll people. They want to see New York."

At the theater, the three of us sat high in the balcony, tapping our feet. In the cab afterward, Debbie discovered that she'd lost her entire doll family. We searched the gutter and the curb in the biting winter wind, the tears glassy on her fine-boned face. We dismissed the cab and climbed back up into the balcony behind an usher: no luck. We left Sid and Mim's number at the theater's lost-and-found.

In the next taxi, Debbie fell into my lap, much bigger than the last time she'd done that. "I want them back, those same people!" she cried. "Not new people! I want those same people back, even though they may have been . . . dropped in the gutter and . . . stepped on, or . . . mutilated, or . . . their hair torn out."

"Oh, honey, oh, sweetheart. Me too." I held onto her and Seth leaned hard against my shoulder and we sat huddled and sniffling in the backseat, the three of us together. There seemed to be only three of us left in the family.

Track C. No remission. Steady decline.

If only I felt myself larger than life, the voice inside my head pronounced as I drove through blinding winter sun after dropping the kids at school. As Alexander the Great did, impervious, collected, integral. After all, these are the days I may look back to as the days of ease and luxury, the days before I began to turn the body from back to stomach at noon. I have shut my mind to it. How can Ted endure it?

Seth would be eighteen before I got his orange room painted. One Sunday I got up and started in. By noon the walls were a beautiful Williamsburg blue with three orange doors and one orange windowsill sticking out.

"Ted?" I called into his study. "Could you bring me up that sandwich I left in the refrigerator? I don't want to clean up my feet?"

"I'm right in the middle of something!" he shouted.

"I'll wait."

I waited.

Finally, he went downstairs and brought up the sandwich.

"Here!" He flung it at me. "Next time, get one of the kids."

"Look, I know it makes you feel bad when I do the physical work —"

"Oh, knock it off!" He left. "You're so irritable!"

That night I dreamed I was in prison with walls that came right up to the edges of my feet.

Work. I finished a ten-page biography of John Cheever one day and started a picture history of ancient Persia due in thirty-five days the next.

In the house, I'd begun to live only in the corners Ted didn't occupy. So had the children. Subtly, a deadly but odorless gas was filling the house. If you don't talk about what's bothering you, you feel dead. I had to get out of the house.

At the post-Christmas sales, I bought cross-country skies. I took the dirt road down through trees boughy with snow and into the meadow.

How beautiful!

The great white expanse, the blue heaven — scenes printed in the memory so early. The meadow lay open, trackless. Beyond it, small hills rose, furry with the pastels of winter. "Winter is the easiest," a painter had said at a reading in a downtown bookstore, "because it's the barest." Maybe she would be a friend.

Six months until we could tell people.

The meadow led to trees and a road and the road ran down to a small river, frozen solid on top, still alive and flowing beneath. Just like me — I stood on the bank and leaned on my poles. The sun shone on the ice and the great quiet of the physical world wrapped me round and said its usual sweet sweet nothing, and I stamped the snow off my skis and headed back.

Yes, the painter might be a friend.

Only six months to go.

"Daddy's worried about his balance problem," I explained to Seth who'd come into the kitchen shouting.

"But he makes me turn down my records!" His eyes narrowed. He'd discovered the Beatles in the way I'd discovered Charlie Chaplin, as a fait accompli.

"He's never liked loud records." I raised the lid of the chicken soup.

"It's not worth listening that way!" He stood by the work counter, hands in his pockets, face red with anger.

"I know. Can you play them when he goes out?" I tossed in the carrots and celery.

"He doesn't go out!"

"When he watches the news?" I added the dill and the parsley.

"I want to play them when I want to play them!"

I poked at the chicken and tried to think of a reply.

"And he never thinks up games or anything like that game we played when Jane came, Evens and Odds."

Single mothers are terrific at dinner games. I put the lid back on.

"He's tired, with the balance problem. It makes him tired."

I felt lost in unmapped seas whose every direction seemed perilous. I didn't want to talk with either child against Ted or even about Ted. I wanted to provide a light tone but also to talk about the sickness. What to do?

Ted was turning into a saint about the illness. I must tell him how lonely I felt, how separated by responsibility, how oppressed by work. If we talked, maybe we could be together again.

"Ted?"

"Just a minute." His slow getting out of bed and his slow walk to the bathroom. One night would he fall?

His return. "You want to hear the latest? I can't press down the keys on my typewriter anymore."

"That's awful."

"So what was it you wanted to say?"

"Nothing. I forget."

"Why don't you go for a checkup?" Ted remarked when I turned forty-five.

"I'm fine!"

"You never know. Go."

We'd stopped taking health for granted.

"Nothing's the matter," I told the doctor. "I'm just tired."

Standard tests showed microscopic blood in the urine, and he ordered a kidney X ray and a bladder exam. It could be kidney stones. It could be cancer.

I didn't tell Ted.

My medical books reassured me: neither cancer nor stones seemed to fit. I leaned back in my plastic chair between the stacks of papers and the baskets of laundry. I felt fine, but I'd read that spouses of the sick often got sick, they often got breast cancer, especially during the first year.

I lay my head on my arms. Cancer of the bladder? My own body betraying me! This is what Ted felt all the time.

If I was sick, how would Ted manage? How would the kids get to school? Get raised? All those lessons. You win some, you lose some. It's not a bowl of cherries. How to bake a cherry pie. I love you. I couldn't be sick. I wasn't sick. The doctor was conservative, that's all.

In three weeks I knew it wasn't stones, but my bladder test kept getting postponed. On the day my mother's furniture was due, I was still waiting for the results and Seth had strep.

The van pulled up, and the movers were just beginning the struggle of getting the piano up the porch steps when Seth came to me at the door.

"I think I have appendicitis, Mom." He stood holding onto his side, looking white, frightened. "I want to go to the doctor. I want to go right now."

Anything could turn into a balance problem.

In the emergency room, a surgeon let Seth lie on a leather chair in a waiting room rather than on the paper-covered cot in an examining room. We didn't yet have full coverage in Massachusetts, and that simple stratagem would save us fifty or a hundred dollars.

Oh, Dr. Schweitzer, you darling.

Floors below they might be working on my bladder cancer results. If Ted had multiple sclerosis and Seth had appendicitis and I had cancer, who would take the car in for the oil and lube tomorrow?

Seth looked at me while the doctor pushed at his belly.

"Just gastric is my guess." The doctor resettled Seth's shirt. "Nothing to worry about."

"You were good, kid, to ask to go. Right on the ball." We stepped out through the door.

"You can die in the night." He didn't need to hold my hand on the way out, as he had on the way in.

"I know. The girl behind me did in first grade."

Back home the movers were waiting, and I reached for my checkbook to pay them when the phone rang.

"This is the doctor's office, Mrs. Greenstein. . . ."

I didn't have bladder cancer!

I didn't have anything, I was fine!

I closed the door on the movers, on the last of the ten months of moving. The house was freezing.

"God, Maggie, I was so worried. "Ted put his arms around me in the kitchen. I stood very straight because if I leaned against him he might lose his balance.

We turned up the heat. We celebrated with a roast beef supper. Our Victorian house was complete. We were, sort of, successful free-lancers. Everything was as if in the land of Normal and Upwardly Mobile. Ted was just doing a little less and I a little more.

"Let's play hearts!" Ted called out and we dealt out the cards and lit a wasteful winter fire in the fireplace.

Later, in my study, I watched the moonlight on the fir trees. Above me late snow gathered on the sloping roof that we could, if you didn't count the mortgage, call our own. The wolf, however, had slipped past the lock and lived inside the house.

## Chapter 6
# Changed Dependencies: Mama (or Papa) and Baby

————◆————

Consider this scene: It's morning in Manhattan. A woman pushes a man in a wheelchair to a curb. She hails a cab. She opens the cab door. He stands shakily and she helps him in. She folds up the chair. She stashes it in front. She walks around the cab and gets in beside him. Do you think:

    a. Oh, the poor man.
    b. Oh, the poor woman.

————◆————

He or she grows weaker, you take over, nobody sees. Whatever he can no longer do, you do. At first you were horrified together, now you move apart. He loses control over his body. This scares you and you begin to watch very closely. The loss of control over his body frustrates him and he tries to exert control over yours. His wish is your command. That was great when you were scared that he would die and you were saving a life. It pales. Most everybody identifies with him. "How is he doing?" they ask. "How is she doing?" At first, that's all you cared about, too. Now you sometimes wonder why no one asks about you. You feel like the agent of another person. You start to feel that you don't exist.

It's a double whammy. First you become a superman or superwoman; then you become invisible. This is the nugget that underlies the sick-and-well marriage and all future chapters here. Although you didn't notice when the situation was acute, you now see that the sick person is number one and you are number two.

Let's start with superman or superwoman. The work load doubles and the energy to meet it halves. How hard this gets depends on how and in what ways the sick spouse is disabled. Does the sickness require nursing? Are there young children, too?

Laurie and Bill raised two children in upstate New York and put them through college before Bill became disabled. At forty-eight and fifty-eight, they planned to "thumb their noses at the empty nest," but then Bill got congestive heart failure. He had to quit his job. The next year doctors gave him a diagnosis of chronic obstructive pulmonary disease. Instead of having fun, Laurie deals daily with Bill's troubled breathing and shortened life span. Bill does a lot: he handles his illness; he supports Laurie emotionally by encouraging her to jog and by leaving small presents on her desk or short notes in her gym bag; he helps with housework, including some laundry. Laurie wants so much to maintain their male and female twosome — she never wants to sink to her being a nurse and his being a patient. Because of Bill's prognosis, Laurie maintains some of the acute emotions.

> Although I work full-time as a secretary and have my moonlighting job as a typist — a real godsend — I've had to become more self-sufficient and self-reliant. It's hard to do this and still preserve my husband's self-esteem . . . to make him feel that he is needed, that his manhood is in no way diminished, and that he is still a contributing partner to our marriage. I must make constant, if low-key, assurances about it. . . .
>
> You learn to cope by yourself because there really isn't time to dump your troubles on your best friend's shoulder. The lawn has to be mowed again, the chimney needs cleaning, the woodbox is empty, that leak in the roof isn't going to get any better — so you work like hell and you don't think too deeply. . . . You cannot go to the man who has always been a solid rock, a pillar of calm, and say "Hey, I'm burned out, I'm exhausted, I'm tired of all this sickness and making compromises and accepting limitations and staring down death every damned day."

In Houston, it has been five years since Lisa's diagnosis of Lou Gehrig's disease and she's still walking, holding onto the walls and furniture. Like Laurie, Tom handles the acute emotions and the double whammy at once. In their three-story brick house painted white and surrounded by oleanders, Lisa mothers the two grade school children as well as she can. Tom has cut back on his work as an account executive to be home more. Even though he has help, he responds to and handles the constant alert that fills the house:

> We have help to clean and to iron, and a young neighbor comes around to help out a couple of days at dinnertime. I'm here evenings and mornings. I go to see the kids' teachers. We go on camping trips. I even bake cookies. I always did a lot with the kids, even before. I've always worked hard and played hard. I'm just now deciding what I can really do. I've come to the conclusion that I cannot go on doing everything I have been doing.
>
> I represent four clients, billion-dollar businesses. They've been incredibly supportive, partly because they've made a big investment in me and I'm very good at what I do. What I've been trying to figure out is if it's wise to have my office phone installed here. I just had it put in, but I find it very difficult. My work style is energetic and I've just about decided that I can't possibly do everything and also deal with the emotional problems of my children and my wife and myself. It's very hard, the kind of toll the illness takes — a constant emotional unrest is the best way I can describe it.

Laurie works full-time, moonlights, and keeps the home with help from Bill. Tom works full-time and cares for a lot of things at home. In many cases of chronic illness, two salaries shrink to one.

If it's the wife who's well and works for wages, this can mean substantial downward mobility for the whole family. In 1985 the median income of married couples where both worked was $36,431, according to the Census Bureau. If just a male worked, it was $22,622; if just a female, only $13,660. The well wife returns from her statistically lower-paying (sixty-four cents on the male dollar) job to perform from thirty to seventy hours more of homemaking a week. There's less attention for everyone and less money.

If it's the husband who's well and working, he doesn't have it much easier, although the family may. He loses his wife's wages and some, if not all, of her thirty to seventy hours of unpaid home labor. He must fill in. He must satisfy children already made anxious by their mother's sickness. Often this demand comes when he is just getting ahead in his career. "The husband of the chronically ill wife must forge on in his career at the same time as he assumes the physical work of managing the house and the emotional care of the children," says Dr. Myron Eisenberg, chief of psychology service at the Veterans Administration Center in Hampton, Virginia (see Appendix B). "It's easier if the children are grown, because the husband will probably be in a more nurturing mode and able to care for his wife." There's less attention for everybody, but not such a big drop in income. The well husband may even manage the situation by greatly increasing his work load and hiring help at home.

If there is an economic fall, it's sure to bring emotional ramifications. How does it feel to slip down the economic ladder? Katherine Newman, assistant professor of anthropology at Columbia University, found out by studying four groups of downwardly mobile American families. In 1986, Dr. Newman spoke at Columbia's Dean's Day about her study, which will be published in book form in 1988 (see Appendix B). One of her four groups was divorced women. What happened to those women reminds us of what happens to families where the husband is sick and the wife well.

Women divorcing at mid-life and living with teenaged children in suburban homes felt fear and a terrible loss at watching their families fall apart. They went out to work. Their teenagers withdrew, ignoring and resenting the mothers from whom they were separating anyway but who could now no longer afford to buy them the sweaters or the skis. Some women moved to less affluent neighborhoods where their adolescents felt isolated.

Younger divorced women were partially reincorporated by their parents through gifts of money. Their preadolescent children still loved Mom and helped out. These women sometimes veered into the New Age dream of surviving spiritually on the cheap, while their children dreamed of restoring themselves to their former affluence.

A second of Dr. Newman's groups also rings bells with sick husbands and well wives. Managerial men who got fired felt humiliated and unmanned. They had believed in the meritocracy. It had betrayed them. They felt like failures and grieved for years. The rest of the family grieved too. They labored to maintain middle-class appearances, just as we downwardly mobile families of the sick do. They turned inward and cut ties with friends whose activities were too expensive. With the sick, the expense isn't always in money but sometimes in simple energy — we can't keep up. Dr. Newman's fired men couldn't go to their families for money, that would have been salt in the wound. Their children sometimes forsook the work ethic and began to believe that what mattered was contacts. The children wanted to get rich quick. And they hated seeing their fathers home all day doing women's work. The children didn't know if their reduced status would be permanent. Like the children of the sick, they felt confused. What is real? What permanent? When will I move back into the class whence I sprung? The children of the fired men ceased mourning only as they grew up and into their own lives.

---

## GET READY TO FALL

It's best to fall out of the middle class and into the arms of unemployment, Medicare or Medicaid, or a college's financial aid office with your records in order. You might adapt a cardboard box with hanging files. Keep names and phone numbers of all doctors, hospitals, agencies. Keep your bills, receipts, notes. Even your parking receipts and gas may be tax deductible or insurance refundable. Is day care deductible? Photocopy all letters concerning money; date everything, including the year. Every day, people discover that medical policies would have covered something for which they have no record. Once you get a system set up, it pays you back. Laurie puts it this way:

> After you've recovered from the initial shock of diagnosis and come to the realization that you are the Responsible Party, there's one thing you must learn to do — keep accurate, complete files. This means medical, insurance disability, any paperwork that pertains to bills, hospital records, prescriptions, correspondence. Your files are go-

ing to be voluminous. Get acquainted with the fine print in the Medicare booklet. Make copies of everything you submit to insurance companies for reimbursement.

———<◈>———

Now let's look at the second part of the double whammy. Many chronic illnesses bring an almost inexpressible exhaustion. The sick lose life force. They require their own attention all the time. One patient kept candies by her hospital bed for the nurses because she was too tired to give them any other attention. "I was so tired," she says, "so sick. I didn't care what anyone else needed. It didn't matter. But I wanted the nurses to like me, because any one of them might help me to stay alive."

Ah, poignant, sad. But we mustn't look at anything too long from the sick person's point of view. Their point of view is what's so dramatic. It enchants. It sucks us in. Nothing else seems to matter. And that, in a nutshell, is the second half of the double whammy. The well spouse doesn't count.

In Georgia, Kathy describes the often recurring self-orientation of the sick. Her husband is bedridden. She dresses both of them each morning, brushes both their teeth, hoists him via a lift from bed to TV chair, then goes to work to help support him and their two young children.

> I am tired of being the well one! No sympathy from a sick partner — none at all. I often think he thinks the way I did when I was pregnant — no one but *me* in the whole world was pregnant. He feels he's the only one in the family with an ache or a pain.

There's an apples-and-oranges split in the marriage with chronic illness. The sick spouse (apples) has one experience and the well spouse (oranges) another: the sick spouse, being in the more critical position, always comes first. In Houston, Tom analyzes it:

> Things that are good for the patient aren't necessarily good for the others around. For example, everybody encourages the patient to stay as active as possible and not to give in. But something is needed for the peace of mind of the spouse, too. I needed someone to be in the house so I could relax when I was at work. Otherwise, I would worry all the time about Lisa falling

down. She didn't want anyone. It's hard to argue that your own peace of mind is important. So you don't. So you worry.

I'd like to talk about the illness and Lisa doesn't want to. There's the natural denial of the patient and that is aggravated by the health community. Everybody wants the patient to give it the good fight. The sick are in a performance position. The denial becomes frustrating to the other person. It gets debilitating.

In Pasadena, Francie describes the second half of the double whammy. She took an unpaid leave from her fledgling magazine and stayed home to handle the crises that seemed to appear every two weeks during Eric's first year of kidney failure. Short of money, she picked up small cash teaching an editing workshop. Here she describes how not mattering, not being seen, feels:

I'm so lonely — sexually, emotionally, physically, intellectually. A crisis is better. In a crisis, you get attention. . . . I miss the office so much. The cliché is true — that the smallest things make a difference. If your husband's very sick you can go whole weeks without being touched or looked at or talked to. At home, nobody perceives you! Then that first day on the campus I was walking along and a student said hello to me. I existed! It was worth the commute just to hear my name spoken.

If the family with chronic illness hasn't been widely studied, the alcoholic family has, and the resemblances open our eyes. The drinker always comes first. Everything in the home radiates toward him or her. If we think of the family as a butterfly mobile — an image once suggested by the renowned family therapist Dr. Virginia Satir — then the alcoholic's family can be imagined as a mobile in which he is the lead butterfly making constant and unpredictable motions. This is how a pioneering therapist for alcoholic families, Sharon Wegscheider of Sioux Falls, South Dakota (see Appendix B), describes it. The alcoholic's wife or husband and the children adjust to the drinker's every unpredictable move. For them, there's no rest. No balance. Physically sick husbands or wives dictate the mobile's movements too, Dr. Wegscheider suggests, though their shifts will be more predictable. In fact, Dr. Wegscheider sees the butterfly that represents the physically sick parent as being stuck to the wall. The other butterflies hang forever in altered, uncomfortable positions.

Another counselor for alcoholic families say that "alcoholic families are remarkably alike and resemble bereaved families, or those with chronic mental or physical illnesses." This is former jazz musician and drug abuser Michael Elkin, who became a family counselor in the Boston area and wrote about what he saw in the alcoholic family. Elkin is insightful about the nondrinking spouse, sometimes casually called "the enabler" or the "co-alcoholic." A current idea is that if the wife didn't allow and make up for the husband's drinking, he would bottom out and stop drinking sooner. Elkin takes a close look and describes the process whereby the alcoholic's wife gets caught in her own efforts to keep the ship afloat. It's very similar to what happens to the chronically well spouse.

As Elkin has stated (see Appendix B), he once told participants in a workshop to pretend they were sifting the résumés of applicants for the job of alcoholic's wife. What characteristics would they want? Replies divided into two directions. One bunch of characteristics clustered around supercoping; they were as follows: skilled at organizing; competent at many tasks, able to learn fast; unflappable; diplomatic; lots of energy, indefatigable; skilled administrator; good at crisis intervention; works to 120 percent capacity; strong sense of right and wrong. In other words, when the alcoholic fails to function, his partner must function to the point of overfunctioning — she generally becomes what's seen as a workaholic and a nag.

Don't think anyone loves her for it.

The second bunch of characteristics clustered around self-denial: skilled in nursing, caretaking; able to defer gratification; resilient; able to bear pain; loyal to others; puts others' needs before her own (best managed by losing touch with her own); never asks "What's in it for me?"; can do enormous work for little reward; defends her own boundaries, perhaps by developing symptoms herself — of migraine, obesity, or depression; has low self-esteem, is very dependent. In other words, the alcoholic's wife gets cornered into becoming the passive-aggressive saint whom everyone avoids.

Sound familiar?

Elkin is quite clear that there's precious little escape because the job molds the worker. An alcoholic's wife who has been on the job five years, he maintains, will possess all these traits with variations according to ability, cultural programming, and availability of resources — such as money. Nonetheless, "any long-term female co-alcoholic will fit the pattern." And that's not surprising, Elkin holds, because the job is so demand'ing that it offers few options in handling it. "When a job is sufficiently demanding, it will describe the person who holds it."

How shall we de-saint ourselves? How shall we keep from playing nurse to patient? The job, as Elkins says, is the job. Still, we can try what seems to hit home to de-Mama or de-Papa and de-saint ourselves. How can we try to untie the knot of the double whammy?

*Loosen up on sex-role division of labor. Check to make sure division isn't really a power play.* One of Edward Speedling's heart attack couples, the Ambrosios, came to grief on this shoal. Mrs. Ambrosio felt woman's work was woman's work. Mr. Ambrosio played a more flexible game, but he played for power and control. It began before he got sick, just after he retired. Like downward mobility and alcoholism, retirement brings situations resembling our own.

Mr. Ambrosio was bored and started to get up at dawn to make the coffee or mop the kitchen. Mrs. Ambrosio hated that. Although still a legal secretary, she loved best her earlier days of homemaking when the kids were small. Here she'd shone. She'd loved setting the table and cooking supper. Now she felt stupid and deprived of her domain. She set her alarm to beat her husband up. He set his earlier. The contest ended when his heart attack stopped him.

In the intensive care unit, Mr. Ambrosio ceased fighting. Back home, he did everything his wife told him. She read poetry to him and chose his clothes and told him how and when to eat. Flexibile, Mr. Ambrosio took up painting and ceramics and even hooked a rug. But his thoughts were still on power: "You are a little person," he told Dr. Speedling. "You are sick. . . ." Mrs. Ambrosio felt very competent again. She salted down the sidewalk after a frost and felt happy, remembering herself as a young girl on her parents' farm, feeding the chickens.

Then Mr. Ambrosio began to mend. The emotions of crisis that bring us together lessened and they entered Phase Two. Mr. Ambrosio didn't want to be the little person anymore. He told his wife that she nagged. They began to set their alarms competitively again. "I'm up at first light now," Mr. Ambrosio told Dr. Speedling proudly. "She screams at me. I say 'right' and go ahead and do it." Mrs. Ambrosio remembered that her husband's doctor had told her he'd never change a tire again. She felt she must watch to make sure he wasn't overdoing. He got sneaky — this is the defense of the powerless, says Dr. Speedling.

Bit by bit, when Mrs. Ambrosio wasn't looking, Mr. Ambrosio sawed a big branch that had fallen in the yard. She didn't notice it, but she did catch him plastering a ceiling. Was she taking good enough care? She had to double her efforts, as he doubled his. She decided to stay at home and watch him more carefully. She stopped seeing friends. She stopped going out. Shortly after, she was hospitalized for a nervous breakdown.

If you've always had a strict division of labor, try throwing it out.

*Are you playing Mama or Papa more than you need to? Is your spouse playing Baby more than he or she needs to?* Sickness is a great place to compete without showing it. Who's calling the shots, the Mama or the newborn baby? There's terrific power in each role. Sigmund Freud referred to an infant in a baby carriage as "His Majesty, the Baby". An old Algonkian riddle asks who has more power than the chief man. The answer is his baby son.

Which is more powerful? Mama/Papa? or baby? There are tyrannies of weakness just as there are tyrannies of strength.

If you overplay Mama or Papa, you make the sick person feel more anxious and more disabled. You give the sick one permission to curl up and sit. It's tough to hold the line. One woman's husband suffering from postpolio syndrome needed to be suctioned. The nurse told the wife she'd have to do it. She refused. "Not me," she said. "He'll have to learn to do it himself."

And he did. It took months. She watched him struggle with the movements until he mastered them. She was able to insist because she, too, had learned to suction herself as an adolescent when she had polio. Most of us haven't endured the sickness of our spouses.

But how practical is it for us to sit still while a spouse struggles with discomfort and courts danger to carry a dish to the dishwasher?

Very practical. Just not very comfortable.

84    MAINSTAY

Yes, we will sit anxiously until the deed is done. But if we offer and he or she accepts with relief, we have sanctioned Baby. The sick one would have been more adult to ask for help. Yet the disabled don't always know what they can do until they try. Okay, then — let them try, fail, and eventually ask for help. We don't have to be there forever noticing and offering. If we are, we're playing Mama.

We must move in the direction of letting go, even if it means sitting with our mouths shut and listening for the crash.

*Too much automatic aid can foster too much cohesiveness.* "Over-functioning and under-functioning are two ways of responding to stress," Harriet Goldhor Lerner, Ph.D. (see Appendix B), senior staff psychologist at the Menninger Foundation, explains from her office in Topeka. "When trouble hits, one person will cope by putting energy into focusing on or worrying about others rather than worrying about himself or herself. Another person may respond to stress by not coping or by inviting the other to take over. The dilemma is that the two approaches dovetail. Things can get very polarized."

Naturally, the situation of the sick and the well fits in all too neatly. "But people, including the chronically ill, have a great capacity over the long haul to manage their own pain and deal with their own problems," Dr. Lerner maintains. In chronic illness, "the well spouse can learn to care for the other person without becoming overfocused on that person and without sacrificing herself or himself. It's a difficult balance and requires continued work. It is important, for example, that the physically well partner keep on telling the sick partner his or her own problems. Too often the physically well person may think 'Oh, I don't want to burden him or her with that.' And sometimes the sick person doesn't want to deal with the well person's problems because he or she has got enough to deal with. Here the well spouse might say 'I'm not asking you to deal with it. I'm just needing to talk about it.' This kind of exchange would help to avoid the false polarity that the physically sick partner has all the weakness and the well person has everything together. If you can share *only* your competence with a sick partner, that partner will have a harder time identifying and utilizing his or her own strengths."

Maybe your husband is the kind that doesn't talk much? "Hang in anyway and try to keep things in balance," Dr. Lerner says. "The challenge is to stay in emotional contact, not to distance yourself on the one hand, or to become overly intense and reactive on the other hand. There's a tendency to go to the extremes of distance and fusion. That middle balance is hard to achieve when you're dealing with a chronic illness because you're dealing with a chronically high level of stress. And it's under stress that people tend to get polarized."

So, kvetch, now and then.

*When the sick spouse takes charge, show appreciation. Don't criticize.* Laurie, the moonlighting secretary, says she never forgets to tell Bill how much the notes in her gym bag mean to her, nor how his help with the laundry matters — she never criticizes his folding.

It's tougher than you think. Monitor your own responses for a day.

*How can you get the chronically sick spouse to give to you?* Ask directly. If he or she gives, don't go overboard. It could be so delightful you find yourself lying on the metaphorical couch, shouting "Help me some more!" Keep it small. Keep it continuous. If he or she doesn't respond to some small request, examine the request to see if illness or fatigue really does prevent it. If not, point this out. Keep on asking.

*Set your own limits.* Practice saying no. It doesn't have to be so drastic as refusing to learn to suction. Francie refused to chauffeur Eric to his hemodialysis if he didn't arrange with her the night before.

*Assertion: the middle path.* Assertion marks the middle path between the sufferer's stance and the bully's. The silent saint says too little, too late. When she can't bear it any longer, she blows — ineffectively. The aggressor says too much, too soon — also ineffectively. These extremes may fit the well/sick spouse twosome rather neatly. The sick may bully a passive helpmeet. Or the well may bully a passive and sick mate. One or both of you might profit from the short course in assertion doubtless offered at a local YMCA or listed in the local newspaper. Or you can read about assertion. (See Appendix B, Lange.) Learn where politeness ends, what your own rights are, how to get rid of martyrish or aggressive lessons learned as a child, and practice, practice, practice.

*Cut the work: reevaluate rituals that involve work.* Francie says, "Thanksgiving we are going to friends down the street. I'm not going to do Christmas. If somebody wants to shop and to cook, okay. You learn that you have to shut down and conserve your energy. You just have to. If you go, it all goes."

*Cut the work: most housework boils down to the relocation of objects; strip down.* Possess as few objects as possible. You may realize only a twenty-dollar profit on your annual tag sale, but the real savings come in reduced work load.

*Recognize the natural effects of always taking second place.* Once upon a time, a woman bore a daughter. In two years, she bore a son. The daughter loved to play softball. Whenever the family got up a spontaneous backyard game, the son would run to the yard, shouting "I'll bat second! I'll bat second!" He knew his place. Imagine him years later, married.

That's us, the well spouse.

Always taking second place makes you feel angry and competitive. Compared to that of the sick, our pain is not so painful; our joy must be mitigated; our fear is not so fearful; shhh, we mustn't alarm him.

Now the fact is that we can't rush into the bathroom ahead of our spouses. We can't go to the movies if he or she isn't feeling well. A sick spouse gets first choice every time.

Really, every time? Think again. It won't hurt him or her if you get to choose the TV programs. It won't hurt if you go to the movies alone. Choose some small ground where you'll have first choice, first place. Shake off the habit of second-placeness.

Look what happened to Abel.

--------<◆>--------

## (Keep Your Sense of Humor Department)
## PIN THE TAIL ON THE ILLNESS

Are you feeling weighed down by the work load? As if you'd faded into nothing? Don't blame it on your husband or wife. Don't blame it on yourself. Stick it on the illness. Really, stick it. Buy some of those brightly colored gummed circles at the stationer's. Draw a big circle somewhere and label it "the sickness". When you feel one of these emotions, stick on the right color.

GREEN: jealousy at being number two
WHITE: a fear of not existing

RED: anger at his (or her) not taking responsibility
BLACK: being deprived of pleasure by too much work

When you get done you will have a flag of Italy bordered in black, but I didn't promise you a how-to. All I can give you is a companion guide.

# Chapter 7
# Wars
## Without Roses

Ted got stoical and cheerful. The books said that MS gives people a false cheerfulness — as well as poor judgment, lack of insight, and irritability. Was it poor judgment when Ted called me names in anger? Wouldn't anyone with insight know I wasn't ratty? The amphetamine he took daily to loosen him up could be making him irritable, too. Or was I a rat? How to sort it out?

My mother grew up in a house with fighting and vowed never to raise her voice to her husband. So I grew up in a house without one single overt argument. I learned silences and inflections, I learned tiny rebellious alterations in manners. Ted grew up among squabblers. He learned to defend and attack and to forgive and make up. As secondborns, we both assumed the other person would take charge. So what were we always fighting about — as we learned the difference between an oil burner and a furnace or where to buy bread on Highfield's main street? Personal history? The rigors of marriage? The stress of illness? Or just oil burners and bakeries? I couldn't think fast enough during the fights to sort anything out. I began to live alone, to live at the side of my husband rather than with him. In my dreams I saw Ted sitting, criticizing me. Finding fault, interrupting.

I dreamt of a coffin in the shape of a long, thin bird with wings too small for flight. I dreamt I was in prison, walking with a man who was in for murder. We walked oddly, lagging behind the others. I didn't sleep a lot. In the double bed Ted's leg jerked in hundreds of small tremors per hour, part of his neurological decline. Before the diagnosis, I'd kicked him softly to stop it. You don't kick a sick man.

If I ran out of wine or butter seconds before guests were arriving, I couldn't ask Ted to go to the store. Nor the children: they were on the last page of a book; they had a friend over for the first time in weeks. I telephoned guests to bring me the butter. They never asked why. What exactly did they notice? If only we could level with them!

Weekends Ted read the entire *New York Times,* Seth played Dungeons and Dragons with one or two boys who liked it, Debbie tried to make new friends in our neighborhood. I did the bills. I clipped the bushes. I made calls for the social calendar. I took rugs to be mended and picked up chairs from caners. It seemed that the rest of the family lived in the middle class and I in the working. How could I complain? Ted had a new symptom: he had to lift his right leg into the car with his hands.

At breakfast he could raise his spoon okay with his right hand. By suppertime, he could lift it only with his left. He taught himself to shave, to sign checks, and to type with his left hand. The problem became editing: how to make pencil notes on copy when you can't make your fingers go. He walked to town to get a haircut, stopping on benches to rest. He drove himself slowly to meetings of the Historical Commission. Tuesday afternoons, I drove us to the meeting of local writers. No one ever asked why I drove. What did they notice? Despite his troubles, Ted pulled in his fifteen thousand dollars that first year. I fell about ten thousand short on mine.

Family to the rescue. Susan had already delivered an electric typewriter. My mother sent money for occasional housecleaning help. When the snows cleared, my brother flew in from Minneapolis and raked thirty bags of sodden leaves, hosed down the inside of the garage. Mel and Doris sent checks for family entertainment. The first few we actually spent on movies and ice cream cones and going out to dinner. After that, things got too tight. My mother drove up at Easter and took us to a restaurant: how shiny everything looked — crystal and silver and waitresses in black aprons.

Susan and Matt brought an air conditioner from their garage and Matt placed it in the bedroom window. It was only April, but summer could be dangerous.

"You should file for unemployment," Susan remarked in the light-filled living room. Amazing how sunny a room remains, if you never get to the curtains. Susan ran a small social service agency. She knew things.

"I'd be embarrassed." Ted sat in the chair with his right arm resting in his lap.

"You deserve the money." Susan lighted a cigarette. Good thing Seth wasn't around to tell her how nicotine poisons the body. "You've got to file within a year."

The cars in front of the ranch-style school began honking, but Debbie wouldn't get out of the car. Her New York surgeon had taken away her glasses to see if her eyes would keep straight unaided.

"You don't understand." She kept her hand on the door of the ancient Buick. "I've worn them all my life. They've always been on my face — between me and — the things. I feel funny without them."

When I picked the kids up after school, she ran to the car — her delicate face freed of metal and plastic.

"Was it okay?"

"What?"

"Without the glasses."

"Oh, sure. Jennifer invited me to her ballet recital. Where's Seth?"

We sat in the auditorium and looked up at a stage full of boys and girls in tutus and leotards.

"Which one is she?"

"Jennifer has long blond hair."

We searched the stage.

"All the girls up here have long blond hair," Debbie concluded rather wistfully.

"Is her name on the program?"

We perused our programs.

"All the girls up here are named Jennifer," Debbie pointed out.

"Do you like it here now?"

"It's okay. But when I grow up, I'm going to live in New York. I'll have my kids at Susan and Matt's house in the country and then I'll move to New York."

"A good plan. I'll visit you. Dad and I," I corrected myself, "we'll visit you."

Forsythia bloomed in the driveway and we shed our jackets.

"We are now leaving the Greenstein compound," Seth droned from the backseat, as if he were speaking into a microphone. "We are bound north northeast to the concentration compound. We will be locked in and drilled on inconsequentials. Give nothing but name, rank, and serial number."

We passed the YMCA. Did he feel as trapped as I?

"On the left you may see the Children's Mission, where they sometimes try to make approaches to us. Take your last breath as we pass. You will not get another breath until recess, at which time you must protect yourself not only from them but from your teammates as well. Give only name. No rank, no serial number. After recess there is nothing until returning to the Greenstein compound, which is better than some if your sister does not eat all the cookies."

They ran out at the school, their backpacks open, their sneaker laces untied. Maybe it was just spring fever?

Ted was never irritable with friends.

"How does he look?" I asked Sid and Mim as we walked down the dirt road, down the hill, under the budding trees, round about through the meadow, with the four children running ahead. They'd rented a station wagon and brought Stan, who was sitting on the porch in his wheelchair while Ted took a nap.

"Frail." Mim's brown hair was going gray at the temples. She and Sid were dressed in brand new white pants and Topsiders: they dressed for the country as I dressed for New York.

I felt fat in my old jeans. I'd finally cut my long hair and when I looked in the mirror I saw my aunt's round face.

"He's remarkable." Sid's stride was as long as Ted's had been. "Just remarkable. I can't believe how good-humored he is."

New leaves uncurled at the tips of the branches; the river ran high. Back home, I served them mustard chicken and asparagus on the porch. Later it rained, a wonderful engulfing rain that drenched the lilac bushes around the porch. We sat in the darkness and talked. Sid was doing a TV show on the gentrification of the Upper West Side. Mim's agent was trying to land her the Hers column in the *Times.* Stan had bought his condominium and was angling for a rental brownstone.

"This is just how I imagined you both." Stan turned his wonderful grown-up face — he so resembles the men of my father's generation — from the darkness in the yard, from the invisible, felt trees. "It's wonderful to be here."

As I set out the berries and cognac, I realized something. "We didn't feel entirely here until you came. Now you're here. And so are we."

Ted looked thin in his summer shirt. He actually weighed less than he had in college. We were surviving on the unemployment he had put in for and won. They talked on. Ted made jokes. He would hear only cheer, false cheer. Ted and I were living two different lives. I skittered along the ground, a fallen kite. I no longer had what Sid and Mim had — what the novels called a heart's companion.

"What's the matter, Maggie?" Stan turned his face to me. Even on the dim porch, Stan noticed. "The life just went right out of you."

"She's tired," Ted answered quickly for me. "That's all."

When they left, Ted slept for two days.

Down in the cellar I looked for the screens Matt had stored behind the grindstone from my father's family's farm. My father used to help out the family of an alcoholic. "They can't depend on him for anything," he explained, intent on giving me the complete moral education. When the wife died, I laid eyes on the husband at her funeral and told my father the man seemed perfectly fine to me. "Oh, most everybody comes through in a crisis." My father smiled in the intolerable way of adults. "The time to check back is in a couple of months." My months were turning into years. I went to see Nellie.

Her house smelled of oil paint and turpentine — smell of art, smell of freedom. Her kitchen had a round table like mine and on it a white bowl filled with lemons, just lemons, perfectly balanced, perfectly spare, perfectly lush. Her overalls were striped with paint and her blue-tipped fingers spattered with colors. Her black eyes grew lustrous with tears as she spoke.

"He left two years ago, went off with her. I cried for a year. My boys told me to stop. They said it was boring. They said they couldn't do anything for me. They said it made them feel helpless. Then Barney left home too young and I don't even have his address. And Nat got that poor girl pregnant and suddenly where there had been a family of four with a mother and a father and two curious, wide-eyed boys, there's just me. I cry every morning for an hour before I can get to work."

"Oh, Nellie." I told her a bit about my life but couldn't mention the disease until August. She and I are exact opposites: she emotes and suffers publicly. I try to keep calm and kindly. Yet we both get up early every day and get to work. We work hard. We tried to help each other.

"You need to learn the middle ground," I told her. "You've got to give a dinner party."

"You don't complain enough. You should let go and get mad." She handed me her bowl of raisins and sunflower seeds. "You should cry."

"I wish I could give you my strength, baby." Ted's father put his arms around Ted after listening to him make his slow unsteady way down the back stairs into the kitchen: a short older man with his arms around his tall, wobbly son.

Doris went to bed with a headache. It hurt her to absorb Ted's decline at each visit. I hurried up the stairs in the front hallway.

"Where's Maggie?" Mel asked Ted as they sat in the living room below.

Up in the bathroom, I unscrewed the broken screen window that I'd forgotten. It had to be repaired that weekend, before mosquito season. Ted didn't want me to ask his parents for help.

Mel stood in the bathroom doorway.

"You should have asked me."

Mel and I put in the rest of the screens and Doris made supper.

"You're wife's working too hard," Mel told Ted over the salad.

"Oh, Maggie's a workaholic," Ted replied, trying to get the peas on his fork with his left hand.

"Actually," I said tersely to Ted later under the brown

bedspread, "I'm not a workaholic. Actually, I'd like to spend the day getting a massage and eating at the French place. My husband would suggest we take the kids to the steak house. I'd teeter about on my high heels and wear gloves to protect my three layers of Apricot Golden. And when the band struck up my husband would extend his arm and say 'Let's cut a rug, baby,' and then we'd —"

"Bitch!" The children would hear. "You're so self-centered. You think of nothing but your own body. You do nothing but complain!"

One complaint was more than Ted's.

"My friends tell me I don't complain enough."

"I wish I could help." Ted stood on the porch as Debbie and I carried her trunk down the steps and into the car. Because he was watching us, we moved faster than was comfortable. Then the three of us piled in for a ride through woods to a Girl Scout camp on a lake.

"Pretty, isn't it?"

"Leafy." Ted's voice sounded a bit off.

I parked in the coolest place and snapped a photo of Ted and Debbie, head to head. Both their eyes were slightly crossed; both wore sweet smiles. Then Debbie and I hefted the trunk over a rutted path to her tent, slowing down when we were out of sight of the car. I cut my farewell short because Ted might be too hot in the car.

"There's something wrong with my left eye," he announced as I pulled away. "My good eye. It feels grainy."

At home he washed it.

The next day he couldn't see out of it.

"A Miltonian mist." He made too light of it.

"Call the doctor."

"When Johanna leaves."

"Call him now."

"I'll wait to see if it gets better."

We sat on the porch in the scent of lilies of the valley, while Ted made jokes with his visiting cousin.

Growing hysterical, I finally unraveled to Johanna in the kitchen. "I'm worried about his reality grasp. The books said MS brings euphoria, *la belle indifférence*. Do you think this is it? It does something to the forebrain neurons. I guess it's like being on a drunk. What do you think?"

"He's got to call the doctor." She came fresh from the real world. And among the Greensteins, women take charge directly, skip the wiles.

Monday the neurologist put Ted on cortisone. Tuesday Ted stood in the kitchen and covered his right eye with his hand.

"Hey!" he called happily. "Everything's okay now! I think I can see the refrigerator!"

"What do you mean, think?"

Wednesday he could really see it. He could also make out the big letters on the cereal box. But he couldn't read his manuscript.

Although in most cases MS blindness clears up in a few weeks, Ted's neurologist suggested he go into the hospital for intravenous ACTH treatments to hurry recovery and reduce the strain of waiting.

July, not August, but we had to tell Seth the whole truth before Ted went in.

Seth was sitting in the living room on the dark couch pushed into the bay window, reading *Dune Messiah*.

Ted sat on one side of him and I on the other.

Ted lay his left hand on Seth's knee. "I am going into the hospital for a while because there's something wrong with my eye. I can't see."

"You can't see?" Seth's lips got tight.

"Just out of my left eye. I can see fine in the other. It's connected to my balance problem. And my balance problem . . . turns out to be connected . . . to something else."

"What?"

"It's . . . called multiple sclerosis."

"Oh." Seth's lips began to move. Tears rolled down his cheeks. He maintained a deadpan look. Then he simply lowered his gaze and pretended to read.

"Wait a minute!"

"Don't you want to hear more about multiple sclerosis?"

"I know all about it." He labored to keep his voice level. "Jerry Lewis is raising money for it."

"That's muscular dystrophy, sweetheart!" We put our arms around our son, who didn't want there to be evil in the world or orphans or nuclear war, who informed guests that it would be better for them if they didn't smoke.

He cried. We held onto him and onto each other. It was the closest we'd come to a real emotion for a long time.

"It's good to cry."

Our own dry eyes met over our son's head: one future down, one to go.

I took Ted to the hospital and left to shop for food. We could tell everybody. It was such a relief. Nellie first.

"That's awful." Nellie put her paintbrush down and led the way to her kitchen. "When you said you were going to the hospital twice in one day I thought maybe you were a drug addict stopping by for your methadone. But you're not the type."

Home to telephone. One of the men from the writers' group had thought Ted drank too much. One of the women had figured something was up: "He's unstable on his feet." Someone else knew exactly what it was: "My uncle has MS and they walk just the same."

After the phone calls, I found the washer jammed. Its white top looked smooth as it gurgled, and I lay my head down on it and finally cried a few tears. I couldn't afford more.

So the long denial ended.

At the hospital, the ACTH was helping Ted's eye. I blew dry my short hair and got into a skirt I'd found for $9.99. Not bad.

Ted handed me a letter from his hospital bed. "Mail this, will you, with an envelope?"

"Who is the gorgeous woman you see before your eyes?" I kissed him goodbye.

"You."

"Am I all there?"

"You're all there."

"With your left eye, am I?"

"Move back. Stand there. Perfect."

His vision returned but not his flexible focus. He had to hold books and paper at a certain length to bring them into fine focus.

In the elevator I unfolded the letter. "Dear Tim, Only now do I realize that I have been denying my illness for two years. Only now do I begin to confront the reality of it. To do so means to become either stoical or very depressed. So far, I've been only stoical and that's too painful. I don't want to do it anymore. I am going to try to be less stoical. Maybe I'm headed for a crash of some kind. But here in the hospital hooked up to my hormonal drip, everything, including my vision, seems clear. And I want to tell you how much your friendship means to me."

I got tears on the paper. Ted was entirely in touch with reality. I need hardly worry about brain function.

"That was beautiful," I called him from the phone booth. "And true."

"What if I get really depressed, though?"

"You'll get really depressed, so what?"

Back from camp, Debbie sat on the same couch, her legs covered with mosquito bites, her hair unwashed.

"Blind? You mean you can't see? You're looking right at me."

"Well, I can see a lot better now." Ted adjusted his glasses. "But I have to go back to the hospital tonight for another intravenous shot. It's related to my balance problem. I have a . . . disease. It's called multiple sclerosis, a long word."

"I know that word!" Debbie looked relieved. "I know a lot about that!" She jumped up.

"Where are you going?"

"To get a book."

Her long legs vanished through glass doors, up the stairs. We held hands and waited, but we dared not talk.

"It's okay!" She ran back down and handed Judy Blume's *Deenie* to Ted. "Read this."

"Scoliosis. This girl has scoliosis, dearie. It was sweet of you to get the book, but what Daddy's got is sclerosis. It's different. Multiple sclerosis."

"Is is bad?" Tension appeared in her narrow forehead.

"It can be," Ted took hold of her hands. "Some people have lighter cases and I hope to be one of them."

She threw herself into his arms and cried.

"Whatever happens," his voice wavered, "we're together."

"I don't . . . want anything . . . to be . . . wrong with you!"

Our eyes met over our daughter's head. It was finally over; all the futures were down. Maybe now we could get really depressed and then put the pieces together.

But we never did get depressed together. When Ted's vision returned, so did his cheerfulness. We did a little talking, but when the talking ended, the illness remained. August came and Ted filed against the private insurance company. Debbie started fifth grade at the redbrick school a couple of blocks away because she wanted to walk to school with her friends. Seth started junior high downtown.

"How's Ted?" everyone asked. On days when three of the Greensteins would be lying abed with sore throats or whatnot and I would be carrying trays and running to town to mail out something for a deadline, they'd meet me in the street and ask, "How's Ted?"

"He's okay!"

"How are you, Maggie?" One of the writers from the Tuesday group ran into me in the supermarket.

"Me?"

"Yeah, you. My brother had leukemia. I know what it's like."

He put his arms around me and we hugged. How sturdy he felt, how strong. I could lean.

"I'm awful."

"I know," he said, as we stood beside the *Familia*. "It sucks."

An editor at the new *Savvy* remembered me from the old days and wanted to send me to Chicago to cover a conference on stress. "Go," Ted said. "It'll be good for you to get away." Yes, I thought. Back to that part of me that's free of sickness.

I found myself sitting next to a wisecracking Californian. "Francie Nichols," she introduced herself, "stress personified." She had started up her own women's magazine in Los Angeles. We got together afterward and ordered up a bottle of chardonnay. Instead of finding the nonsick part of myself, I sat in Chicago and told poor Francie the whole story of the last two and a quarter years.

"I'll tell you what you need," said Francie, who had raised a brother after her mother died. "You need psychotherapy and you need to find a lover."

"I've had too much therapy already and I don't want to ace out on my husband."

"Then what you need is another drink." She poured me the bottom of the bottle.

"I'll talk. You keep quiet." Ted tried to smooth the fingers of his right hand flat against his thigh. We drove past January fields to the Social Security office. Jimmy Carter, Susan had told us, wanted to help. This was a kindly society. Ted could qualify for federal disability insurance. The private insurance company was still investigating our case. Forget shame, did we want to lose our house?

I sat wordless and watched Ted turn himself from a successful self-employed writer into a recipient of federal funds.

"Okay, I'll submit you for a disabled and let's see what happens." The social worker stapled the papers. "And we'll put in to the state for a word processor. It'll probably be a Radio Shack. If we take you, you won't be able to net more than four thousand dollars a year. More than that," the social worker instructed Ted, "and you lose your monthly check."

"That was the hardest thing I've ever done." Ted sat stonily on the way home. "You don't know what it's like."

"That's right, I don't. What's it like?

"Can't you tell what it's like! Don't you see?"

"Well, maybe now you can finally write the life and times of Pericles, just as you've always wanted." I, too, resorted to false cheer. It offered the least resistance.


"Radio Schlock, I call it!" Ted shouted sometime later at the innocent repairman in the city where we'd driven with the word processor bestowed upon him by the State of Massachusetts. It was a first model of a new line. It was a lemon. On it and on its repairman, Ted finally vented publicly the rage he felt against his own faulty body.

"Who do you think you are, to treat me like this!" he shouted over and over as he pounded the counter with his left hand. The right hand curled up against his chest.

# Chapter 8
# The Chronic
# Emotions

S ix months pass. Or four years. You move from the
acute emotions through the double whammy to the
chronic emotions. The younger you are or the more disabling
the illness, the quicker you move. Somewhat contrary to the
acute emotions, the chronic emotions force people apart.

"In some ways, the chronic illnesses are harder on the
spouse and family than the acute illnesses," says Boston
physician and psychiatrist Dr. Peter Knapp. "The chronic
illnesses are less hard in that the person you care for is alive.
But they are harder in the long sacrifice, the adjustments, the
constant dealing with ambivalence, and the continuing struggle
with the feelings — you get adjusted and then you sink down
a notch and it all has to be reworked and rethought and
readjusted."

Exactly.

Here, from the well spouse experience, come our own
descriptions of the chronic emotions. Don't worry if categories
overlap here and there. You may not have all these emotions.
You may move slowly through them from start to finish or you
may dip into the more intense ones first. You may fall in and
out. It depends upon your own makeup, your family history,
your spouse's response to the illness, and the illness itself. The
first cluster bears some resemblance to the acute emotions,
although it lacks the promise of an end point; it also character-
izes the double whammy.

# THE CHRONIC EMOTIONS

## They Pull People Apart

CLUSTER #1

*Mostly Sadness*

SADNESS: "[We've] I've lost so much."
GUILT: "He's sick. I'm well."
TRAPPED: "Is this it, forever?? [I want to stay. I want to go.]"
LONELINESS: "She's so withdrawn! She never notices me."
JEALOUSY: "He gets everything the way he wants it!"
ANNOYANCE: "I'm doing too much! What's she mad at me for?"

---

### SADNESS

Psychologists think of sadness as what you feel when you either fail to get what you want or when you lose what you love. Emotions may have evolutionary use — after all, they organize us to act, they move us toward things with curiosity or aggression and away from things dangerous. Dr. Jerome Kagan, clinical psychologist and professor of psychology at Harvard University, has been known to say (see Appendix B, Izard) that when the Homo sapiens toddler's fear of strange objects fades and he begins to explore the surrounding forest, sadness may keep him from wandering too far from his mother or other familiar elders. He doesn't want to lose what he knows and loves.

To become chronically ill is to lose yourself as a healthy person: you grieve. To be married to someone ill and to watch a man or woman you love suffer means you mourn. You mourn the lost marriage, the lost family, the suffering of the mate, and your lost self — the one who could feel dependent, who could ask to be indulged, the lighthearted you. And often with chronic illness you mourn a lost or reduced sexuality. Since this is so seldom understood in the literature or by professionals and so hard for well spouses to discuss — yet so much on their minds — we'll focus on it here.

## (Tears of Joy Department)
# THE LAUGHTER OF PAIN

"And now for my last question," the eager interviewer says to the well spouse by telephone. "What about your sex life?"

The man at the other end just laughs and laughs.

The mildest loss is of what we might call cultural sexual identity. Miriam and Daniel enjoy a happy sexual relationship — only their cultural sexuality is threatened. At thirty-nine, Miriam watches Daniel, who has a painful post-polio syndrome; they're both watching television:

> This is what's hard, me in my Naugahyde armchair, Daniel lying on his mats, the egg crate mat, the Thinsulate mat from L. L. Bean, the extra large pillow in Indian cotton. Pill tin in front of him, small bright square of orange paper on which he's keeping track of his seventeen Percodan, his three or four Valium. We're watching the commercials on TV for "Christmas for him" — chain saws and drill bits and screwdriver sets, all the things the man in your life would like, the announcer tells us. Daniel would love them, only he can't sit at his workbench anymore. He does beautiful dovetailing and oil finishing and yet little by little, this, too, is being taken from him. I memorized these lines from *Middlemarch* when I was studying for my Ph.D. exams. "If we had a keen vision and feeling of all ordinary human life, it would be like hearing the grass grow, and the squirrel's heart beat, and we should die of that roar which lies on the other side of silence." I thought I knew what they meant then, but I didn't. I do now.

The next level involves a more physical loss, that of joyful, free, uncomplicated sexual activity. Here fits the fear of returning to sex after surgery or a heart attack. Martha Lear describes it in *Heartsounds*, her book about the four-year sickness and eventual death of her husband Hal. This is their first sexual encounter after his initial heart attack.

It seemed crucial that he not know how scared I was. Lying there silently, as though my mind were on my pleasure. Watching him in the half-light that came from the bathroom, seeing the fingers pressed so slyly against his carotid artery, wondering what the pressure told him. Feeling his rhythm, the contact so sweet, and hearing him breathe heavily like that, and wondering if it was okay or too much. Then feeling his body go still. Was he all right? Did I dare ask? . . . It would be dreadful to make him feel like an invalid here, of all places, in the bed. One wrong word and I might ruin it, erection gone, impulse gone, confidence gone, goodbye, and maybe for good.

And yet it might be even more dangerous to say nothing. For his body was in motion again now, and what if he was feeling pain, denying it, pushing himself to perform?

"Do you want to rest a moment?" I whispered.

Wrong. He made a sound like a sob and fell away from me, and we lay silent, not touching in any way.

Where there is intimacy but the inability to engage in full sexual activity, longing develops. Here Laurie the moonlighting secretary describes what she and Bill have lost:

I'm going to get up from this desk in a minute and help my husband out of his clothes and into his pajamas. I'm going to put some little foam cushions on the incipient bedsores because he's so exhausted when he goes to sleep that he doesn't move much and his skin is pretty tender from the medication he has to take to keep breathing. And I'm going to move his oxygen tank closer to the bed because the tubing doesn't quite reach from the chair where he spends most of the day. After he gets somewhere near to what passes for comfort, he'll reach over and squeeze my hand and we'll both remember doing a lot more than squeezing hands. And we'll tell each other that there's a lot more to love than whole-hog lovemaking. But sometimes I get so lonesome for the familiar loving. . . .

Perhaps the next level of pain comes when intimacy itself erodes, disrupting the desire for sex. This pulling apart may stem from the sick person's needs. "People with chronic diseases often engage in sex less frequently," attests Dr. John Rolland. "Those individuals often have less desire. There's pain. There's fear. And their energy is down."

And sometimes the well spouse may pull away if he or she

hasn't been getting much attention from a sick person who is depressed and angry and self-involved. Intimacy requires full give-and-take. A husband says of his wife after she had undergone extensive chemotherapy: "I wasn't repulsed by her. She didn't lose all her hair. She wasn't mutilated. Still, I didn't have much desire for her. Because of the intimacy questions. They are more key than the illness."

At the next level, some people are repulsed by the effects of their partner's sickness. Alzheimer patients may desire sex in a way that appears subhuman to their partners. Parkinson's patients may get turned on by the chemicals of medication rather than by those of emotion. This may be fine for the patients, but it is tough on the partners. Lack of intimacy plus problems like these turn off the well spouse.

In her mid-thirties, Janice is a suburban New Yorker married to a man much her senior. Not long after the kids were born, Walt received a diagnosis of Parkinson's.

> When we were first married I couldn't get enough. Walt came from a pretty nonnurturing, nonaffectionate family, and I spent a lot of time readier than he was. I never dreamed the shoe would one day be on the other foot. You know, people look at us and all the sick from a distance. They think, 'I bet she's dying for it and he can't function.' But it's not that way. When I look at his tremor, the way he's not gotten dressed, perhaps, or shaved, all day, when I remember how he's shouted at me, I . . . well, I lose it. I don't feel attracted to him at all. There was one whole year when I went ahead, I tried. I forced myself. Afterwards, I would feel so resentful. I would feel violated. That's when I asked him to go into marital therapy.

In therapy, Walt told the doctor he would leave Janice if she continued to turn him down. Janice was cold, he explained. He'd had it with her coldness. When Walt calls her cold, Janice wants to kill him. But she couldn't tell the therapist any of this with Walt listening. It *would* kill him. Janice knows that Walt's threats aren't real, that he just needs to prove himself now more than ever. She keeps on trying to respond. "When I can get to a certain point physically, it's okay. I can remember him how he used to be, I can blur out the details. I can manage."

Janice lives in constant sorrow over the loss of her sexual partner, even though he's right there in bed beside her.

Last, we come to the effects of long-term inactivity. If either partner ceases to function sexually, the other may "put it in the deep freeze," as Dr. Domeena Renshaw, who surveyed the 151 impotent couples, describes it. That's what happened to twenty-six of the wives in her study. They gradually lost all desire for their husbands, relating this loss to years of futile struggle to achieve coitus. Eventually feeling rejected and sexually unattractive, these women had begun to avoid even sexual play in order to "prevent frustration."

"If one has been turned off sexually," Dr. Renshaw says in a phone interview from Chicago, "it's extremely painful to turn back on. It takes a lot of energy to put one's sexuality in the deep freeze. Getting it thawed out again is hard. There's fear and hurt. Trust takes time to build. It takes testing over time. You ask yourself if this person will respond to your needs. Will he not reject me? Will I let my feelings come out of the turtle shell again? It's very hard.

"I've lectured in Sun City about sex and aging. One time an agonized question came from a woman in the audience: 'What do you do if you're trapped in a cage with a husband who has Alzheimer's?' I thought she had tremendous courage to speak. It was clear she had suffered a great deal. It takes a long time for Alzheimer's to be recognized — I guess we can follow a golf cart around without all our brain cells. It's especially hard for a woman of her age because she's been trained never to make the first sexual move. I suggested a vibrator because it's not as destructive to her own value system as seeking an affair would be."

A vibrator may provide sexual release, but it doesn't offer a whole lot of intimacy or equality as a sexual partner. We are still talking about loss.

What happens to well spouses when they deal with health professionals about sex? Plenty of doctors and psychologists don't mention sex and are relieved when patients fail to discuss it, too. They do occasionally acknowledge that a person who has to diaper a spouse may find it a sexual turn-off. I've never heard them extend this to brushing your husband's teeth. When pressed, they tend to fall back on "'sexual intimacy without intercourse" or on "more communication" as the viable options. Communication is just what Janice or the woman in Sun City can't possibly manage.

Dr. Myron Eisenberg of the Veterans Administration Medical Center in Hampton, Virginia, is one of the rare health professionals who pays heed to the well spouse's needs. He's aware of how spouses are often treated by therapists. And why. "We therapists work hard with people who've been disabled by spinal cord injury or catastrophic illness to help them develop ways to function sexually. It's very frustrating for us when patients come back and report failure. We may even get angry at the spouse for not practicing the sexual techniques we've taught the patient. We forget that it's really the able-bodied spouse who puts up with the day-to-day problems. It's hard for that spouse to continue viewing the partner in sexual terms when providing daily care — is she a nurse or a wife? We may establish unrealistically high expectations for her. We encourage the patient to have sexual needs and yet we expect those in the immediate environment to provide the support to meet them. Sometimes there's just not enough energy left in the family unit. We need to remember that it's easy for us to walk away at four o'clock in the afternoon. We expect *someone else* to do it. *We're* not doing it."

"Communicating more" generally boils down to the sick person talking. The sick post pleas in their books and newsletters. Here is one, paraphrased: "Just because we're sick doesn't mean we don't want sex. We do! We need reassurance, though. We need to be made to feel attractive. Keep on caressing us. Make love as often as you can. Show us you still care about us as sexual partners."

Before or after we change the snow tires?


GUILT

Shame serves to inhibit socially unacceptable behaviors. For instance, it keeps down aggression toward younger siblings, or the weak. Guilt comes later and involves disappointment or anger with the self for not doing or feeling what the self views as good. Dr. Kagan has pointed out that guilt takes time to develop partly because it takes time for a child to realize that he has a choice.

In a way, well spouses wake up every morning ahead of the guilt game: here we are, we didn't split, we made our choice, we're Good. But where there is inequality and resentment, there will be guilt. Through the day, we get angry at a person in a weaker position. Nothing that happens to us during the day is quite so awful as what is happening every minute in the body of the sick. So how can we be so rotten as to get angry? We're Bad. By evening, we are filled with guilt.

The guilt makes you do things you really don't want to do. This woman's husband has suffered a severe stroke:

> Last night it was so beautiful. I wanted to get out, to get away from the house. So I said I was going for a walk and he made motions to say that I was lucky. He had no such option. Okay, I came back in. I pushed him out in his chair, along the sidewalk. But it was hard and I was too tired.

Laurie doesn't feel guilt as she jogs to keep herself in shape to care for Bill because their relationship is still pretty equal and because his life is in danger and because she knows she's doing all she can. What she feels guilty about is that she might not be able to simultaneously care for her elderly parents. She'd have a choice. But she'd say no to them. One choice weighs heaviest of all on well spouses, as another woman puts it:

> When we go to the emergency room, the doctors ask about resuscitation. When I give a No Code, I feel so guilty. They look at me funny. No paddles, my husband says. I agree, I wouldn't want people jumping on my chest, either. I know I'm doing the right thing, but I feel so guilty.

TRAPPED

One of the most common questions asked of a chronically well spouse who expresses any negative feeling is "Why don't you leave?" This basic choice gets made over and over. Unspoken answers include "I'd feel too guilty" and "The kids would never forgive me." And "I'd never forgive myself."

> When I wanted to quit the marriage is not when he wanted to quit — so that's what made me stick. If I can be honest, another thing that made me stick was . . . guilt. What would it have looked like to family and friends? Wife walks out on man with lupus? I couldn't have handled that. So I stayed.

More expressible answers come out this way: "She'd stick by me." And "I love him."

The truth usually includes the all-pervasive ambivalence that Dr. Knapp mentioned at the start of this chapter: "I want to stay. I want to go."

Here's the image. You and the man or woman you chose out of all the world because you loved and trusted and admired that one are walking in the woods. The one you love steps in a bear trap. He lies there bleeding and in pain. You both work on the trap, but this is long, long ago and far off in the woods and neither rocks nor fingernails are strong enough to open the trap. He's cold. He's hungry. You build a shelter and look for berries. That's one day. The leg rots. His pain increases. It snows. That's one year. It snows again. You plant a few pumpkin seeds and slap a little mud on the shelter. At what point, exactly, do you say So Long, Charlie?

Any moment is too soon; any moment is too late.

Years go by and the fact is, you have stayed. You are there. Are you going to leave now, after all you've put in?

Some do. "There ought to be a support group for those poor bastards," says a man from Chicago whose wife is bedridden. "They must be in the worst shape of all."

Could you really leave? Jill can't decide. She's shared neither house nor bed with John since their four-year-old daughter was an infant. She hasn't forgotten the bone-chilling night that came after seven months of erratic behavior during which John gave her several black eyes and a cracked pelvis. That night he told her he knew she was a spy. Her job was done, he explained, fervently. It was time for her to leave. She got the baby into her snowsuit, hid John's rifle, stuffed the steak knives under the couch and ran to a neighbor's. Today the doctors aren't sure if John is schizophrenic or manic-depressive, but they do believe he has reached a plateau and must live from now on in a very structured situation, remaining protected from ordinary demands. Jill brings him home Saturdays and Sundays.

I made a promise when I pledged my marriage vows and I meant it. If I didn't care for John, it would be easier. But I care very much. I feel no bitterness. I know it's the illness. And he is Lara's father. That's irreversible.

Weekends John just watches television, sometimes with the sound off. He plays the stereo at the same time and sits and stares. He rarely shows emotion. It's as if someone has taken a pair of scissors and cut the emotional cords in his brain.

Lara is the one he responds to the most. He smiles when he sees her. He holds her and hugs her. Does he feel a father-daughter tie or does he just think she's a great little kid? I wouldn't feel safe leaving her alone with him.

I want to honor my vows. I saw a priest about a year ago. He said I could surely get an annulment. It's important to me, staying within the church. But I still have to come to a decision within myself. What will happen to John if I leave? Sometimes he comes to me and says, "I need a hug." Who's going to give it to him if I'm not there? Who'll make him laugh?

My father says that I've never really known the love of a husband who's committed to me. I'd like that. My parents are a very together couple. They hold hands. At mass last week I heard a couple restating their vows after fifty years and I was crying more than their own children were. I'd love a marriage like that.

But what will happen to John if I leave? I don't know what to do. I just don't know.


LONELINESS

The friends who came round in droves have gone home to their own lives. Sometimes they don't come back.

A man from Maine reports:

> We lost friends when Jerilyn went blind — a particular couple we'd called regularly before. They just started seeing less and less of us. They made excuses. And that made me bitter. It was the only thing that made me bitter.

The sick spouse protects himself or herself by drawing inward. There is less talk between the two of you. The man from Chicago who suggested a support group for men who had left their sick wives placed an advertisement for female companionship in the *New York Review of Books* for himself.

> I placed the ad because of the loneliness, intense loneliness. It didn't have to be for sex. If I'd just wanted sex I could have walked into a bar in the yuppie section wearing a Botany 500 jacket. But that's not what I had in mind, a mistress. I wanted a woman to talk to. I wanted female nurturing. People walk into

my house and smell the urine, see the commode, see my wife —
so depressed. It seemed like something to do, a way to get away
without splitting. The ad didn't work. I got a handful of answers
and I took two women out for dinner. One had a husband with
advanced diabetes and the other's was brain dead. It was so sad.
I didn't want to make the lives of either of those women one bit
harder. I'm a man of tremendous energy and I found the
solution to loneliness by increasing my work load. I started
putting in sixty or seventy hours a week and I'm feeling better
now. I'm making lots of money and I can pay for a nurse for my
wife. I'm still immensely lonely, but not like I used to be.

There's also the lost social scene at home. The well wife is too
over extended to give dinner parties. She turns down others'
invitations because of medical emergencies or fatigue. Pretty
soon there aren't so many invitations. Francie says:

After a year nobody invites you anywhere anymore. We had
two invitations for dinner this entire year and I had to cancel
both because of some crisis or other of Eric's. A couple of days
ago we were actually going to some small event, and when I
opened the closet door my eye fell on some dressy clothes. I
hadn't worn them for a year. A terrible feeling came over me. So
I dressed up for this small event and then I started crying.

Sometimes the loneliness comes from not having anyone to
share pleasure with: a woman whose husband had myasthenia
gravis says that when they went on vacation "I went with Max
and he went with his myasthenia gravis."


JEALOUSY

The young Brooklyn sculptor Leah remembers the days before
her marriage to Michael. Although she was the bride, the
newly diagnosed and newly threatened Michael got most of the
attention.

Here was this precious person everybody wanted to hold onto.
I wondered, "Would they do it for me? Would they come to my
funeral?" Infantile, but I wanted someone to take care of me. On
one level, the competition was there before the illness. I always
felt Michael was more charming, more popular, more likely to
succeed. My brothers had been succeeders, too. So there I was,

feeling competitive with Michael because of his tumor, so inappropriate! But he *was* getting all the attention.

Sometimes the jealousy directs itself toward the people out on the street or in the restaurant, the people who can walk without assistance. Or toward the people at the celebration wearing tuxedos, dancing to the music, drinking the champagne — people full of exuberance and vitality. You are holding your husband's hand so he can manage a couple of stairs and noticing that the button on his coat hangs loose, that the coat itself is shabby and that he needs a haircut. But you were shoveling a path to the car and didn't notice in time. May their champagne spill out of its glasses! May their tuxedos wrinkle! No, no. That's petty-hearted and we don't want that. Oh yes we do, sometimes!

### ANNOYANCE

Irritation comes with the increased work load. A well spouse may bear every responsibility from screening the cellar windows through preparing the taxes to buying the blueberries — as well as writing the sick spouse's letters. That's Part A. Part B involves dealing with the sick person's own irritation at being dependent.

And sometimes the sick have nothing but that dependency. It's the only ballpark they can play in. This can drive the well spouse wild. Again, Francie speaks:

> You know what it is? You're presented with feeling murderously angry with someone you know you still love but can't reach. I can't be his nurse or mother. He's so incredibly dependent. I try to get him to take his medicine. He says, "You can't make me!" But when the doctor gives him the medicine, he takes it fine, oh, just fine! I can't force-feed him and I can't monitor him. Yet when he doesn't take it, I can't help but notice — it eats at me and before I know it, I'm hyperventilating.
>
> Eric's thinking about whether he wants a transplant. I have to start the rounds. He has that blind trust the sick have. I'm the one to find out which program, which hospital. The doctor says that the disease shouldn't become your life mission. Hah!
>
> The nurses love him. According to them, he always has a sense of humor. Until I come in. He saves all his anger for me.

"Bitch!" he calls me, after a solid hour of "Shut that window" and "Pick up that glass."

A month passed and Francie assembled the information on the transplant.

I got all this stuff, mounds of literature on the transplant. I left it on his bedside table. So far I've found the material on his bedside table unread, on his desk unread, in the living room unread, in his briefcase unread. We had a screaming fight about it today. I won when I threatened to stab him through the heart in one swift thrust. What do I mean I "won." The pamphlets are now in the kitchen, unread.

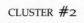

CLUSTER #2

*Mostly Anger*

ANGER: "He's mad at me all the time!" "He bosses me around!" "I'm mad at him all the time!"
ISOLATION: "He doesn't call his friends anymore." "I'm the only one he talks to."
BOREDOM: "Sickness! I'm sick of it!"
HUMILIATION: "It's awful not to be able to buy the kids what they want!"

Annoyance moves, as we've just seen Francie's do, into anger. Jealousy or competition make continual domestic war. Loneliness grows into an encompassing isolation; the illness mushrooms to cover everything; economic decline provides the pincers for the squeeze from outside that completes the picture. The emotions of Cluster #2 spin the well spouse far away from the sick.

ANGER

Years ago I was sitting around a table of writers, all laughing. A young man was telling of a couple he knew where the man was sick and the woman was actually angry at him. "Can you imagine," he said, in disbelief. "She was angry at him for *being sick!*" I laughed innocently with the others.

Recently a woman with arthritis spoke with me about a support group for couples. I asked if the well spouses ever mentioned anger.

"Anger!" she replied. "Isn't that disgusting! How could they get angry at us!"

Easy, that's how. You wouldn't believe how easy. Anger is endemic to chronic illness. You just aren't allowed to express it.

You can call a WASP a WASP, but can you call a crip a crip? You've got to call a crip "differently abled" or "someone who lives with illness." (I drove twenty miles in a snowstorm to a conference with that latter phrase in the title, mistakenly thinking it was a conference for the well spouse.) Sick is sacred. Sick jokes are the sickest. Who would wish the sick ill? Only a creep.

A woman in an airplane put it this way, as we flew over the Great Salt Lake Desert:

> When people hear my husband is sick, they say, "Gee, how awful. It must be awful to think of your husband as sick. It must be awful to look ahead to the future." Well, I don't do that anymore. I take it day by day. This may sound funny, but those aren't the things that bother me. What's hard is living with someone who's angry all the time. What's hard is living with someone who shouts at me when he's angry. What's hard is living with someone who's apt to blow up at the kids without cause. Just when they are trying to help him with something — like handing him a ballpoint pen too slowly, or stumbling over the rug when they're helping him with the trash. They're just kids. I have to step in. That's what's hard. But you can't say that to people. They'd think you were terrible.

Perhaps the evolutionary significance of anger lies in the fact that it establishes submission or dominance, as the psychologist Dr. Kagan has suggested. Homo sapiens needs group rules to be able to work together. Dominance and submission provide a structure for cooperation. The "best man" wins the right to dominate. Eventually, dominants influence the behavior of submissives by threat only. A simple nod suffices.

Illness threatens the sick spouse. He fights to retain his identity against it. Or he may use the sickness as an ally to aggrandize his failing self. He may need his spouse to be his arms and legs or eyes and ears or his secretary and chauffeur. He may give a lot of commands. The very sick give commands just by lying paralyzed in their beds. The well spouse fights for the lost equality, for her own space, for control over her own actions. Yet she feels subordinated to the sick person's needs, and angry. It's a round robin.

For the well spouse, one particularly frustrating aspect of the sick spouse's anger is that few outsiders see it. The sick tend to collect themselves for visitors — doctors, nurses, friends, even extended family members. There's no corroboration of the sick spouse's anger and no one for the well spouse to discuss it with. The well spouse can get to feeling crazy or guilty just for noticing it.

Simply venting anger doesn't change things, as Dr. Lerner points out in her book (see Appendix B, Chapter 6). Anger, she maintains, is a signal like thirst. It means something needs to be changed.

The sick cannot change their condition.


HUMILIATION

Friends offer you money; family ask if you've got enough. Strangers weigh the two of you to make sure you're frail enough or poor enough to receive their favors. As Miriam put it when a social worker came to see if Daniel could still bathe himself:

> "Do you bathe yourself? Can you walk without assistance?" Businesslike questions, asked in a capable, friendly way. But to admit a certain helplessness in areas so natural for others? No, Daniel can't bathe by himself. Yes, he does need some assistance. And not from a county nurse. Dan should be spared the eyes of a stranger, even if she is a nurse.

Joint humiliation brings you together. There may come the day, though, when you guiltily wish to be dissociated from it.


ISOLATION

The sick person turns more inward. The gulf widens. Yet the two of you are stuck together within the four walls, as socializing decreases. Miriam confesses:

People stay away. It's a downer to ask "How's Daniel?" and always hear "He's okay." It's others' perceptions of us that I'm troubled by. I don't want to be seen as these helpless, ailing people. Daniel on his hospital bed, me tending to him. It's an image that's so static, so depressing, really. No wonder people stay away. And I hate for it to be the topic of conversation.

Laurie discusses some causes of social isolation:

We have no evening social life; by the end of the day there's no energy left but to draw breath, never mind a game of cards or a movie. . . . You don't invite the new neighbors back for supper (I used to love to do that!) because you realized the first time you sat down in their house that they smoked. I tried going to a couple of parties alone; it just doesn't work.

Increased physical incapacitation makes socializing close to impossible. Kathy can't manage much for the family now that Sandy is bedridden:

The pain is in feeling closed in — housebound. No longer do we just take off. One of us always must be home and, of course, it's mostly me. No more going out to dinner, no more vacations, no more weekend jaunts. The smallest Scout affair takes logistical planning to make sure we're always covering the bases at home.

BOREDOM

Trivially enough, the real agony of a chronic illness sometimes seems to lie in its boringness. Steve says:

Diabetics have to eat at certain times and Jerilyn gets upset if we go out to dinner at the wrong time, but it gets boring to make reservations for 5 P.M. Once in a while we make an exception. She can't expect that eight or ten people are going to eat at her time all the time. Damn it all, we can break the rule once in a while.

Sickness curtails. It's rather like fanatical religion — blotting out music and art and skiing and just about everything else. To skew the world to one concern limits vision. Those who don't deny the illness may get consumed with it, instead. This serves a purpose: you learn a lot about the illness. But after a while, it's enough.

---·◄◉►·—

CLUSTER #3

*Mostly Collapse*

FATIGUED: "God, I'm tired!"
DEPRESSED: "What's the point?"
ANXIOUS: "What if? How can I? Watch out!"
OVERWHELMED: "I quit. I can't go on."

—·◄◉►·—

The third cluster brings you close to breakdown. This is
depression. This is temporarily giving up. Everybody does it.
Why not? We are helpless in a way. We are hopeless in a way.
For most, it's temporary — a dip into the pit. Even a good
night's sleep may restore us.

## FATIGUED

We falter under the work load.

Often we sleep in beds or rooms with the restless sick. Our
sleep is interrupted by them. Or we are too worried to sleep. Or
we wake in the middle of the night, frightened and in despair.
Or just waiting for the crash.

Like the mothers of young children, we're almost always
tired. "Last week, for the first time in my life," says one
woman, "I didn't dance at the office party when someone
asked me. Dancing is my favorite thing. I was too tired."

## DEPRESSED

Depression, say the psychologists, may be lots of daily or
monthly sadness turned into an overriding mood. When
you've been sad a long time, you learn to expect not to get what
you want. You become depressed. You tend to blame your
failures on yourself. You lose your self-esteem. You lose your
hope. The world won't change. And you won't change. So
there's no way out. Chronic moods become harder to change,
less labile. Sometimes we're too tired to change. Sometimes the
depression is biological, affecting the centers of the brain that
make us want to eat or sleep.

In Houston, Tom has been depressed off and on ever since Lisa's diagnosis of Lou Gehrig's disease.

These five years have been just up and down and up and down. I used to be even-tempered with bursts of energy and pretty sheltered about my emotions, in the way typical of males. I tried to avoid emotional situations and then I found myself in the midst of one. I'd never had a depression before, but once I got it, it became very deep. It does respond to medication. I go on and off medication. It's not abnormal, my doctors tell me, for me to be depressed in this situation.

Lisa has done very well. If she wants to go on a trip or vacation, she uses a wheelchair. She hasn't had depression. Others have told me I am displaying her emotions for her.

When I'm down, it's just incredible. I have to drag myself around. I'm not interested in doing anything. This is the most debilitating thing that's ever happened to me. I think of suicide.

In Pasadena, Francie woke one morning at two. She called at dawn:

Eric and I are both too reduced to struggle anymore, or even care. This isn't a life, it's a torture, a travesty. My spirit is finally broken. Imagining both of us as suicides doesn't disturb me as it would have before. It's an answer to endless despair. It would release the children to go on to their own destinies.


ANXIETY

Chronic anxiety grows naturally out of the fear we've been holding onto since we got the news. "A heart attack," says a cardiologist, "is a frightening experience. I've had people come in with a second attack after twenty years. They say they remember it exactly, everything exactly as before." The fear never goes away for either spouse.

For the well spouse, the fear becomes apprehension not for our own bodies but for those for whom we feel responsible. Steve speaks again about Jerilyn; although of low intensity, his anxiety is at the ready and all-pervasive.

When Jerilyn was blind, I worried all the time if she was home alone. She smoked like a chimney and I was always worrying about fire. I'd be at work and I'd telephone her and it would ring and ring and ring. Then before I knew it, I'd be in the car heading home. She'd be out in the yard hanging up clothes and then she'd be mad that I'd come home.

Once you've had the bolt of bad news, you lose a bit of your trust and begin to find yourself wondering when the tires will shred. Sometimes the anxiety stems from the sense of having no active team members, nobody to fall back on. You stare into the pit and realize for the first time that you and your spouse could be one of those couples who freeze to death by the side of the highway on stormy nights: you couldn't leave your spouse alone to seek aid.

What if you get the flu?

What then?

You mustn't get the flu!

Quick! Hurry! Run faster than the flu!

### OVERWHELMED

By adolescence, we learn to know when we've exhausted all possible solutions to our problems. It's called logic.

Sometimes there's so much logic hitting the fan that we stop struggling.

So there you have the bad news. Isn't there any good? Of course there is. Later chapters will deal with ways to approach some of these chronic emotions. But certain things can't be fixed and sometimes fixing isn't the point.

Robert and Suzanne Massie raised three children, one a son who was a hemophiliac. When they traveled to Russia in the 1960s, Suzanne Massie felt that for the first time she'd found a place where the language of sorrow could be spoken. Sorrow had its dignity among the Russians, a dignity bestowed by war and tragedy. "Among them, at last," she wrote in *Journey* (see Appendix B), their book about their son, "there was no need to pretend an optimism I did not feel. They understood. No words were needed. . . . Is the loneliness so great that you feel yourself floating away ever farther from reality? They will crowd near you, to bring you back, stroke your hand, gently embrace you. . . . This was what I wanted. This was what I needed. Not pity."

Sometimes the best thing is for someone to look you in the eye and say, "Yes, I know."

Then you can go on.

# Chapter 9
# Downward Mobility

We'd exhausted the canon of accepted medicines — speed, Valium, and forms of cortisone. There was nothing left. Nothing clean. Ted refused the blood transfusions I'd heard about. His neurologist suggested injecting ACTH directly into his spinal fluid.

"I had one patient whose wife wheeled him in . . ." The doctor set the atmosphere of hope with me as we sat outside the room where Ted lay absorbing injected hormones. "Afterward, he got up off the table and walked out to the car."

Ted got up and walked out of the clinic with the newly purchased, hand-carved cane that so deeply embarrassed him — just as he'd walked in. The shot gave him a couple of very good work days and that's about it. Ted drew the line there. No, he would not ever look into blood transfusions.

"Stay away from quacks." Blond Angela took my arm crossing Boston's Pinckney Street, its small cars parked triumphantly in what appeared to be even smaller spaces. An uncle of Ted's had died and I'd rediscovered Angela serendipitously at the funeral: years ago in college we'd sat coiffed in our pageboys sewing numbers on the pinnies of the men's ski team, and now our husbands were both sick. Hers had Parkinson's. "Don't listen to anybody. When people first heard about Ben, they gave us all kinds of advice. It's psychosomatic. Eat this. Don't eat that. Laugh a lot. We did it all. We even went to a woman who dangled a needle over his wrist and told him if it swung a certain way, he'd get better. So don't listen. You'll wear yourself out. Save your strength. Established medicine is bad enough. You don't need homeopathic. That's for prevention. Once you're sick, you need Western." And Angela had lived in Wilson House, with the liberals.

Then the letter came from Mel and Doris. Halfway through our second winter, I was finally making curtains. In the dining room, I unfolded yards and yards of rosy velvet that was actually cold to the touch from waiting so long in the unheated hall.

"Look at this." Ted handed me a note and a clipping from Florida. Roger McDougall in England had cured his MS by refusing to eat any wheat or oats or barley or rye: this is called the nongluten diet. There was a picture of him jumping.

"Hey, try it!" I cut happily into the velvet, scissors crunching against the table. I believe! Even though Angela says not to. I believe! Even though the National Multiple Sclerosis Society warns that no diet, including this, will cure MS. You gotta have hope. What can you lose?

"I guess maybe I'll try it."

Diet is clean. It couldn't hurt.

There isn't now and there wasn't in 1980 any shortage of bean sprouts between the Charles River and the New York State line. You want co-ops with grains of rice crunching into dribbles of honey as you cross the floor? You want long lines of tofu takeouts? No problem. I joined the crowds of enthusiasts in the new religion. The food emporiums sold the holy texts themselves, right next to the millet and the pinto beans. In my own kitchen where the sunlight comes stained red, blue, and yellow through the peace dove stickers that the children gave me for my forty-sixth birthday, I practiced the new vocabulary.

There is, apparently, nothing miso soup can't do. One observer credits the radiation-free recovery of a group of Nagasaki victims to miso, tamari, brown rice, and seaweed. Forbidden to Ted was anything that comes in jar or box. You have to make it all. No animal fats, no sugar but raw. Getting a loaf of rice bread to rise remained a mystery to me for weeks.

"What time are we eating?" Inside the house Ted walked without his cane, coming downstairs by hanging onto the walls.

"Aaah. Having a little trouble with the rice bread."

"Are we eating this glop again?" Seth sat reluctantly to his fare.

"You get a burger option, if you make it yourself." I was eating Ted's menu to learn to make it palatably.

A devotee from the vast and pious network eventually informed me how to get rice bread to rise: you don't grease the sides of the pan. The stuff is too weak to get up greased sides. Grease the bottom, copiously, or the whole thick dry lump adheres permanently.

Seth began to love the potato, his first vegetable beyond the green bean; Debbie wrote "French bread" on the shopping list every week in her round hand. Ted and I felt virtuous, as if we'd given up smoking. Here, at last, was something we could do, some way to fight back.

"I'm hungry." Ted tried, but there wasn't enough to chew on, no comforting pastas, no English muffins, no bagels. The diet added an hour to my day. Less time for the kids and Debbie wasn't doing well. "Between you and I," her teacher at the brick school opined ungrammatically at Parents' Night, "I've dropped her out of the top math group. It's all boys, anyway." There was no time for me to take up the feminist cause. All I could manage was to question Debbie on how many thirds of a cup you need to make a cup of rice dough. And her teacher in Manhattan had warned that she wasn't a child to approach dogmatically.

Seth joined the smaller of the seventh grade's two social classes, the Bookies. The intellectual kids carried backpacks on their shoulders and walked together, heads down, animated in chat. The Jocks wheeled off on one wheel of their bicycles, Look Ma, No Books. The two groups didn't mix. This is democracy?

Bookies were careful to avoid Jocks in the locker rooms. You could get hurt. Years later I found out that's why Seth chose to play basketball at the YMCA. I had no time to learn the children's widening hearts — never easy for the working mother, but I'd always managed until the illness grew into a thousand leeches.

We visited a woman who had kept her MS in check by avoiding gluten. She stood easily at her door in ordinary dress in an ordinary ranch house in the wilds of Massachusetts. On her stove sat a beautiful glass teapot contining twigs of bancha tea.

On her kitchen table no salt, no pepper, only an herb mix in a glass jar. In her refrigerator brown balls of miso and on her counter, the wok. Along her shelves, jars of rice in all its white variety. On the appetizer tray waiting for us: some wonderful raisins that turned out to be currants and some unsalted peanuts. In her living room, a fire in the fireplace. Oh, very pleasant. Her husband carried the tray into the living room.

Cured by diet, would Ted's right hand uncurl, allowing him to carry a tray again?

The fire cracked, the currants and peanuts tasted wonderful. It could be sweet, the life of the devotee. I looked at her husband, peaceful, unagitated.

"If only he'd listened before he had his gallbladder operation, he could have cured himself by diet."

"Not all illnesses," her recuperating husband pointed out, "respond to diet. Not even all kinds of MS — it's mostly the remitting." Snowy trees surrounded the house, visible through its serious array of picture windows. Mostly the remitting? Would we be shut out of nirvana? We talked about illness for an hour. There wasn't a single other wellie in the room. I began to long for a Coke and a hotdog.

"Once in a while," the woman remarked at the door, "my husband takes our daughter out for pizza."

By mid-February I had developed a rice bread that Ted and I could eat. Guests choked on it. I made it every other day, sifting the flour six times in my strainers with a wooden spoon.

The kids kept on swallowing the mainstream's burger and bun, only now I knew what it was doing to them. Tears came into my eyes in supermarket aisles when I read the milligrams of yellow dye #5 being offered the innocent or when I simply walked past the sugar and salt and butter of the slower, seepier Nagasaki. The tears were not entirely for the blitz on our planet's health.

The nongluten diet plus the ordinary diet was expensive. Ted's unemployment checks — he'd received seven — and my ghostwriting barely paid the YMCA's modest fee for Seth's basketball uniform. And Debbie wanted a Sony Walkman.

"Kid, you'll have to return this raisin bread." I picked it out of the cart and handed it to Debbie as we approached the checkout counter. "We're over sixty bucks."

"Mom! What about toast?" Her eyes looked slightly crossed

again, and wistful. The surgeon said not to worry, she'd develop a near and far eye like Ted's.

"We've got a rye and we still need baking powder and cornstarch and almonds for . . . Daddy's bread." It was hard not to dump all life's problems on the illness and, therefore, indirectly on Ted.

"I hate rye!"

"Seth likes it. Next week it'll be your turn."

Once, remembering the pies and cakes and hot fudge sundaes my mother lavished on me, I broke. I placed a bottle of butterscotch sauce into the cart. When the kids were helping me unpack at home, Debbie discovered it with joyful shock. She took it into both hands and held it to her cheeks. "Mom! I think something . . ." — she paused to compute an explanation for this impausible bounty — "fell into your cart."

The visits of our New York friends usually began with their bags and bags of house gifts: expensive cold cuts and cheeses from Zabar's, bagels from ye olde corner bakery, bottles of wine. Unpacking, I couldn't help but tote up well over sixty dollars. Their cars weren't rusty and in need of mufflers. Their clothes remained chic, their hemlines in fashion. They reported vacations. To Europe long ago, they were now touring China. And they exhibited, as usual, good health. Good health! It seemed to be another state, blessed. They could lift trays and carry books and walk to the river. And their children looked happy, flourishing. Whatever problems rose in learning or socializing or the body physical were instantly noticed and dealt with by doting Mom and doting Dad. We doted on MS.

Once, after a visit from Sid and Mim and Andy and Grace, I went into the cellar and cried while the day's rice bread rose. Debbie came down. I dried my eyes because it can't be good to have a mom who gets tears in her eyes whenever she sits down. She clumped steadily down the rickety stairs in her clogs and emerged into the half darkness.

"I just feel like sitting in someone's lap," she said, "and crying." So I held her in the porch chair with her legs dangling. We sat surrounded by memorabilia, including the swinging piñata, now dusty and damp.

"What I miss most," she said after the tears, "is picnic time, real time, not five minutes at bedtime. *Be* with me."

"I'm right here, right here." But soon I had to go and get the bread out and more, more.

After a few months on the diet, I felt great. Lighter, more energetic. I even looked better in the long mirror of the bathroom: not bad for forty-six, slender enough now, better color, and with my eyes cleared of city air, I could wear contacts again. Could I find another man? What kind of rat would leave Ted? But there was something to this diet — Ted might improve!

Although he didn't enjoy the food, Ted sat on the kitchen stool with his legs out of range of the stove and invented a little song for the first grain produced by the Neolithic revolution, the perfectly round grain beloved of the ancient Near East. *Oh, Millet! Oh, Millet! Queen of the Grains. You keep away gnats and bring on the rains.* Once he would have soft-shoed to it; now he sat in his gangly layers of sweater. It seemed like home, nonetheless. And it felt so good to actually be helping Ted.

We served our guests rice and steak with scallions sautéed in tamari sauce and wine. When people invited us out, I called to explain Ted's food needs. They loved it. Cooking special foods made them feel they were helping, too. Extreme diets do make you feel wonderfully self-righteous — an honest soldier fighting an evil enemy.

"No one needs to be sick," a young man remarked in the line at the health food store. "Unless somehow he wants to be sick."

"That's not true!" I turned and snarled. I simply couldn't control myself.

He smiled as if my anger were part of the problem.

"Susan?" I hung on the wall phone in the kitchen as I sifted flour. "Can Matt fix the steps of the front porch?" Matt had put in a new back porch and fixed telephones and glued chairs and handled several seasons of storm windows.

"Name the day." Susan did paperwork for Ted and found out about grants and government benefits and invited the kids to Boston and produced holiday meals and encouraged me in my own work: "Just because the illness hurts Ted's career doesn't mean it has to hurt yours."

I didn't tell her there was a balance of $4.65 in the bank. Kind of hard to stretch that for two weeks of food. On the other hand, a missing $115 might come in. Or not. Ted never seemed to know these things. It scared me to be taking over the entire balancing of the budget. Before Ted had wanted to discuss it; now he preferred not to hear how hairy the money situation grew and accused me of worrying about it too much.

But Ted ate so well now, maybe in six months without gluten he'd be better? He fell at the writers' group, barely missing the metal base of the table with his head. He fell downtown coming out of the barber's. But it takes months, the diet.

Ted's being in the house every day got to me. No wonder women go crazy when their husbands retire. I couldn't get away from him or the illness. I couldn't concentrate on the short history of the bathtub while he was clinging onto the walls down the back stairs. This time, the crash? The crack of the head?

"Rent an office," Trisha advised.

"I'll help pay for it," my mother offered.

"Here's one for fifty dollars a month." Ted showed me an ad.

So I rented an odd-shaped, almost triangular room over a hardware store. One window looked toward Seth's junior high, and one morning when we ate breakfast I packed their lunches and one for myself: peanuts and cabbage — none of your dirty breads, etc. "Goodbye!" I kissed Ted as he lay in bed upstairs in the brown flowered room. When we were first married, I'd had a job that began later than usual and Ted had kissed me goodbye in bed, smelling of after-shave and hope.

It was wonderful that first day, wonderful, not to be thinking about Ted, to be existing as myself. Who was that? It had been two and a half years since Ted had been stopped in his tracks. No matter. No more. I was taking action to fix it.

The first day in my office, I hung a potted plant in the window and charged up a space heater at the hardware store because it was freezing in my small, white-walled room. Then I organized files, reread some old published pieces of mine. They were funny. What had happened to my sense of humor?

No matter. No more. Now I'd recovered. Now I'd get myself back. No sickness. There would be no sickness here in the white room with the sunlight and the plant. This would be a well office.

With my jacket on for warmth, I ate my peanuts and my cabbage. Then I put my head down and cried. Here I was, in my own space. And Ted's illness was right there beside me. His cane and his limp and his fatigue and all the other problems were right there. In fact, shouldn't I run down to the five-and-ten and call up to make sure he hadn't fallen? No. Sit. There is no sickness here. But, as in Chicago with Francie, I couldn't shake it off. There would never be a life without it. I would somehow have to grow beyond it, not let myself stop at its enclosing wall.

"Mom! Mom!" Both kids would scream accusingly at me when anything went wrong. Since I was responsible for everything, everything was my fault. Good logic. If the car skidded on ice, if I overshot the budget and we had to drink powdered milk, if I couldn't fix the washer, if there was no money for new jeans, if I burnt the rice — Mom! I labored fruitlessly against their way of dealing with the world. And they seemed sad.

"How are the kids?" Susan's voice came into my ear over the phone. "Do they talk to each other about the MS? Do they talk to you?"

"No. I try. I ask how they feel. They don't say much."

"There's a good family therapist I just heard of, she's got MS herself. She's got kids of her own."

*She* would help me get Ted to telephone the car mechanic or the neighbor with the snowplow. *She* would help me get the kids to clear the table and rake the leaves cheerfully.

Debbie liked the idea best. The day I told her what a mess her room was, she replied with passion: "I can't wait to get to that person where I can talk about my feelings!"

Seth seemed lukewarm. He was playing a solitary round of Dungeons and Dragons in his blue room upstairs. "I don't have anything to say." He was wearing a red plaid shirt like the shirts boys wore when I was in seventh grade, a boy shirt.

How long since I'd seen the kids for fun?

Ted sat in front of his word processor, prints of the art of Greece at the time of Pericles about his room. This ought to be the ideal life!

"I'll go if you really think we need it," Ted answered. "But no more long-term stuff, no more Dr. Miller."

"Don't worry. Blue Cross only pays for ten sessions."

*         *         *

Dr. Thomas's office lay sixty miles away, and I kept the accelerator at 57.5 in order to make her only postschool appointment. At 4:01 on the first day, we drove up in front of what had to be her building, cars swerving around me, no place to park.

"Get out. I'll find a place."

Ted reached for the hated cane and got out. The kids followed. I reached the office some fifteen minutes later. Bonds had already been formed. I felt like a second course. Smiling, attractive, not yet using a cane, Dr. Thomas welcomed me warmly. It was her life goal to see that no child she encountered gave up his or her future to nurse a chronically ill parent.

Good. Mine, too. I'd read in the books that this was a danger.

She asked the children if they'd ever been embarrassed by their father's appearance. Seth sat in his plaid shirt looking sad. He said he worried only that Ted would die. In her short, glossy haircut, Debbie slouched and reported that just before Ted got his cane he was lurching as he walked around the neighborhood and a boy had shouted at her, "You're defective and so is your father!" She'd felt awful.

"Who said that to you?" Ted asked.

"What did you say back?" I wanted to know.

"What matters," Dr. Thomas wisely pointed out, "is that she's talking about it now. How does it make you feel, Ted?"

So we found a way into our lack of know-how for talking over the illness. How verbal we were in the rest of life!

"I guess it's good I got the cane, then." Ted rested his right hand over its curving handle. "If I have the cane, the kids in the neighborhood will know there's something physically wrong with me. They won't think I'm lurching about because I'm a Phantom of the Opera or anything."

Every Wednesday, I kept it at 57.5. Once Seth sat in back with Ted and asked him to arm wrestle. Seth arranged it so Ted won. Once Debbie sat in back with Ted and they made up a poem:

> *My daddy wears glasses.*
> *He has flowers in his ears.*
> *My daddy looks funny.*
> *And he's looked that way for years.*

128    MAINSTAY

*My daddy's a tough guy.*
*He knocks out people's teeth.*
*He has an arrangement with a dentist*
*Who pays him by the week.*

I managed to get the three of them there in time, but continued to arrive late myself. Afterward, we walked across the street to Burger King and bought the kids some regular burgers, no expensive quarter pounders, and a soda each. No frappes. Ted couldn't eat that food. And I couldn't afford it. The trip's five dollars in gas for our high-riding guzzler came out of my weekly ten dollars for personal expenses. I might need a Chapstick or to make some business calls to New York from the booth in the five-and-ten. Sometimes I packed apples for the ride home, but I never got organized enough for the beautiful picnic I nonetheless fantasized for the top of the mountain between Dr. Thomas's office and home.

"No. You can't have the milkshake, just a small Coke. No, you can't have the apple pie." It hurt to deny the children such simple things. I got hungry and grumpy on the ride home. We never reached my problems in the sessions. I couldn't seem to mention them. The prospect of Ted with his cane and this woman with her recent devastating diagnosis sitting in their hesitant postures trying to sort out our life was too much. At times I would fantasize going out for coffee with Dr. Thomas's husband (he'd pay!), who sounded like the saint I loathed to become. In his heart, he might be as seething or as sad as I.

Debbie the eager was getting bored with the regimen. One day when she had a cold, we took Seth alone. Dr. Thomas had Seth draw and label an emotional "pie" for each parent. From this exercise, we learned how Seth perceived us. He let us know that his father was angry, gave too many orders, and shouted too much. He let us know that his mother was too sad.

"I guess," he said quietly, in his plaid shirt, eyes thoughtful behind his glasses, "being sad is another way of being angry and that being angry is another way of being worried."

We three adults looked at each other with tears in our eyes.
It was a wonderful moment.

Seth drew a pie for himself and gave himself a sad slot, too. And a slot called "wishy, washy and confused."

On the way to the elevator, he laughed and seemed happy. Grown to our shoulders, he took our hands. We stood linked together in front of the elevator. It was worth every one of the seven hundred tight-timed miles I'd driven and all the Chap-sticks I'd gone without.

After this, Seth, too, got bored. Spring was coming.

Apparently, they had exhausted their agendas. I hadn't even broached mine. When Dr. Thomas told us we were not a family in crisis and could take a summer break if we wanted, we leapt at the chance. We were a model family. Come back if we hit crisis. We never did. We voted to spend the seven or eight dollars the trip took on the movies or at our own Burger King, and order the frappes. Debbie entered the all-town fifth-grade spelling bee. She had to cue me in as she went out the door, I was so preoccupied.

"Say it."

"What?"

"It starts with *G* and ends with *D* and starts with *L* and ends with *K*, what is it?" She stood almost to my shoulders in the jacket she'd chosen against my advice.

She came back with third place.

Nellie's older son shaved his head in California and became a monk in an Eastern sect.

"While we were getting separated, I was so upset, I wasn't there for him," she mourned in her good-smelling kitchen as I sewed by hand the eleventh rosy velvet curtain panel.

I hung the twelve soft curtains in the dining room and living room windows and stood back. Warm and cozy, soft and relaxing. Seth and I dragged the heavy counter out of the kitchen. The floor man ripped up the green linoleum, revealed a buttery pine beneath, and layered it with polyurethane. This was our home. We were getting somewhere.

And the diet — a few months more and we'd know if it would help Ted.

One spring night I asked Ted to show me on my own body his symptoms, and he did. The right leg, unable to raise it; the toes unable to know when they will rise as instructed or turn under and you fall over them; the right hand not comfortable unless the fingers fall toward each other in a loose fist and rest in the lap, or if you're standing up the whole hand moves toward the chest. Holding the fingers flat requires too much effort, too much strength. The smallest three fingers are numb, and none of them can distinguish a nickel from a dime by feel. The sense of the arm being "my arm" begins about at the elbow.

And that's just for starters.

"God." What was there, really, to say?

The next morning I went out to photograph the dogwood tree flowering with a thousand blossoms. The grass stood ten inches high with maple seedlings scattered throughout.

How could I get mad at Ted for not taking charge of the lawn as he'd promised? For not taking charge of Seth's work on it?

"Must be great," my brother said on his summer visit when we raked together, "to have an office. You can go out to lunch."

"It's great. I'd be dead without it."

Lunch? I couldn't afford coffee out. Ted's twelfth and last unemployment check had arrived. The Social Security office was still considering his disability application. The private insurance company was in its tenth month of investigation. If nothing came through, I would be supporting the family starting July 1.

I was brought up when we called ourselves girls, and girls never expected to support a family. When single mothers do it, they tell the world they're terrified, but I couldn't tell anyone but Jane.

"How do you manage?"

I asked her as we walked to the river with Patrick and Seth and Debbie running on ahead.

"That's when I dropped art history and went to IBM. Get a job. You need the benefits."

"There's no work up here but store clerking and running health food restaurants, and you know what a lousy cook I am."

"What about Hartford? Providence? Boston?"

"Move? Are you kidding? I barely survived the last move. And this is a great town for the kids. Besides, I'd have to make forty or fifty thousand to live in a city, and I barely grossed ten this year."

When I turned the corner onto the pretty street, Ted was standing on the porch. "It's no," he said, as I started up the steps.

I knew he meant the insurance company. He'd signed the application the night before he went into Mount Sinai, two weeks before diagnosis.

"A man came with a check for four thousand," Ted went on. "The four we paid them."

"Why won't they take us?" I reached the top of the stairs.

"Because I'd already seen Dr. Astor."

The two one-thousand-dollar bills I'd slipped under the bars at the hospital in New York appeared before my eyes. Lost for no purpose. It was almost worth it, though, to have Dr. Miller proven wrong. And the four thousand would keep us until I found work.

Debbie turned eleven. I took her and several neighborhood friends to an amusement park for a last childhood fling. Seth turned thirteen and did a nice nosedive into the dining room rug when he opened his grandparents' check for one hundred dollars.

Seth a teenager? All I could think about was how fast the four thousand was vanishing. Yet I missed him, missed him.

Then we were saved. I called home from the phone booth in the five-and-ten next to the turtles to remind Ted to defreeze the burger. That's when he told me that Social Security would allow us $1,079 per month until Debbie was through college.

I watched a turtle try to climb out of its glass dish. "I can breathe."

"Were you really so worried?" Ted didn't worry anymore.

More millet. More rice flour. It takes a full year, sometimes, for the diet to show change.

It turned out that a distant cousin of mine had a distant cousin in the forefront of MS research. When this renowned scientist came east for vacation, he would see Ted and give an opinion. Mel and Doris were north, and they drove Ted to the doctor's summer home on the Atlantic. Ted telephoned exultantly from a seafood restaurant.

"I just ordered a popover!"

"Your diet!"

"He says forget it. He says if I were his brother, he'd tell me to go on Imuran."

"Isn't that a dirty drug?" It could hurt platelets. Do permanent damage. Could it cause cancer?

"They monitor. He said to try it for six months or a year and see."

"Didn't he think the diet was good for you?"

"He said my life's bad enough. He said I don't need to torture myself with a diet like that."

"Does Blue Cross cover it?"

"No. But it's just pills, not awfully expensive."

Imuran wasn't part of the canon then. We were out of accepted medicine, out of Eat Right, and into Dirty. I couldn't believe it, so fast!

"Okay, okay, good news! Enjoy your popover!" I wasn't going to shepherd him as the last generation's wives did: stand over him saying no ice cream, no butter, no caffeine. He was grown-up. It was his decision.

Part of me rejoiced: another hour in my day freed up for paid labor! Maybe even to see the kids!

"Come on, kids, we're going shopping! We're going to buy French bread and pasta and cakes!"

# Chapter 10
# Fighting Off the Gurus

---◆---

WHAT TO SAY WHEN SOMEBODY IMPLIES
THAT YOUR SPOUSE IS MAKING HIMSELF OR
HERSELF SICK
BY WRONG THOUGHT OR WRONG ACTION

a. Have you yourself recovered from this same illness?
b. Unprintable
c. Unprintable
d. Seen any good movies lately?

---◆---

From the acute emotions through the double whammy and into the swamps of the chronics, and now before we climb out, here come the mosquitoes. They're everywhere. They sting. They've been flying around since the bereaved and ailing Job sat in sackcloth and ashes at the gate of healers in his ancient city. "It's your fault," his friends told him. "You didn't do it right. You're not right with God."

Here in the New Age we don't pin illness on faulty relations with the Almighty so fast — but we do look deep into ourselves, into our adrenal glands and into our immune systems, and come up with the same reply: "Aha! You didn't do it right."

Are mind and matter so different? Will and being? Chemical

and electromagnetic activity? This intricately complex question surfaces in new forms every generation. A hundred years ago researchers showed that specific "germs" or microorganisms (bacteria, viruses, fungi), not some miasmic cloud of contagion, brought illness. Yet at the turn of the century Sigmund Freud hypothesized that invisible, immaterial emotional conflict could cause certain diseases, such as hysteria. How do psyche and soma interact? In 1929 the physiologist Walter Cannon described (see Appendix B) "the sympathetic response," or what today is called the stress response. One branch of the autonomic nervous system named the sympathetic branch prepares us to meet danger by accelerating heart rate, moving blood to muscles, opening respiratory passages, and increasing breath rate — all changes that allow us to move arms and legs fast enough to fight or to flee. The stress response simultaneously inhibits the internal, vegetative processes of peristalsis, stomach contraction, digestion, and sexual arousal — all activities that enable us to sustain our individual selves and reproduce our species. Too much or too constant a sympathetic response, however, as Cannon showed, can lead to such ills as peptic ulcers (ask your nearest air traffic controller) and colitis and high blood pressure.

Nobody gets through the day without stress. Life is stress. Stress causes a reaction in everybody. Will stress hurt you? Maybe. It's probably genetic which organ system, if any, might weaken or misfunction under extreme and constant stress. If the lungs fail to function optimally, asthma may develop. If cartilage and joints begin to change, one of the 110 forms of arthritis may appear — that is, if you accept the Weakest Link theory. It's an easier theory to accept than Specific Personality theory.

According to this latter hypothesis, illnesses may arise in part from one's own personal history and patterns of social behavior. As one section of this loosely aggregate theory goes, people who appear outwardly strong and aggressive while secretly craving to be cared for may develop ulcers. Another part of this many-faceted idea suggests that time-driven people may worry and hurry and compete their way into heart attacks. Lately, there's the Cancer Type.

For instance, in a book called *Getting Well Again* (see Appendix B), Texas oncologist Dr. O. Carl Simonton and his psychotherapist wife, Stephanie Matthews-Simonton, present earlier commentators on the Cancer Type and then describe this type as someone who puts others' needs first, someone who has trouble expressing negative emotions, and someone who wants to look admirable before others. "Consider," the Simontons advise cancer-stricken readers, "what underlying needs were met by your illness: relief from stress, love and attention, an opportunity to renew your energy. . . ." They suggest that instead of receiving these desired benefits through illness, the patient try to find them through other avenues. (Stop a minute to consider the implication of that train of thought.) And they advise that cancer patients take an active stance toward fighting the illnesses within their bodies by imagining their white blood cells in combat against cancer viruses. "You might picture the cancer as broken up hamburger meat and your white blood cells as large numbers of white dogs coming in to devour the hamburger."

Even though the Simontons may be intending simply to involve the patient constructively in his own progress and to activate his fighting will, the implications of such statements sometimes bear unwanted fruit. That is: if we have made ourselves sick, we ought to be able to make ourselves well — if we try hard enough. Although the Simontons don't exactly make this claim, it is hard for the lay reader not to infer it.

It's not just the Simontons. The You Can Take Charge of Your Health philosophy flourishes in gyms and health stores across the country. What if you're sick — seriously sick — and can't make yourself well? Or married to someone who can't?

If it's the latter, you may get angry. You may think that your spouse could get well by doing more this or thinking more that. Yet you know he or she tries so hard! So you put the lid on your angry suspicion. Then you feel guilty. Just when you've settled your guilt, you read another new report: white cells do respond to stress. During the excitement of splashdown, white blood cell activity of Skylab astronauts slowed substantially. Under the stress of bereavement the white blood cell activity of men in a study at the Mount Sinai Medical Center in New York slowed for four months after their wives died. If psyche and soma are so interrelated, couldn't your spouse get better by eating differently or jogging more, by ignoring ambition or ventilating anger? The next day contradictory reports emerge: tests on mice and rats suggest that stress can also enhance immune activity. Stress can be good for you! Still other tests show no relationship between attitude and recovery from illness. You don't know what to think. What's the real story?

To add confusion to confusion, when physiologists speak of stress they mean such things as extreme heat or cold, viralinvasion, or dehydration. Psychologists mean the loss of someone you love or a threat to self-esteem, or powerlessness. Psychotherapists mean conflict within your personal history. Nonetheless, physicians agree upon and recognize a class of illnesses called the auto-immune illnesses. These appear when white blood cells turn against the system they normally defend. Among these illnesses may number rheumatoid arthritis, lupus, thyroiditis, and myasthenia gravis. If your spouse has one of these, are you going to get mad? That'll help a lot, won't it?

Is he bringing this exacerbation on himself? Why doesn't she stop eating that ice cream, it's bad for her heart! If only he could voice his feelings, his arteries would unclog and his cancers unknot! Of course, you could monitor the ice cream. You could monitor the emotions, you could . . .

Remember that double whammy: if you take charge and bully your spouse into a diet of brown rice and so forth, you are playing Mama in spades. Your spouse may very well resist and take to sneaking or sabotage and play Baby in revenge. Remember Mr. Ambrosio out in the yard sawing sneakily at the fallen branch? Your spouse will be down in the kitchen at midnight looking for the whipped cream. On top of increased conflict, you'll have all that shopping and grating to add to your already massive work week. You'd be thrilled to do it if it cured your spouse. But will it? Mental changes in the sick spouse's attitude may require less of the well spouse's time than cooking changes, but do they really work once illness has affected body tissue? Is your spouse going to feel even more inadequate and depressed if Think Right doesn't work? Will your spouse turn the blame inward?

"The whole notion that proper attitude can cure cancer has negative implications for many patients. When they don't get better, many start blaming themselves on the assumption that their attitude or will were inadequate," says Barrie Cassileth, director of psychosocial programs at the University of Pennsylvania Cancer Center. In 1982, Dr. Cassileth began a study (see Appendix B) of 359 newly diagnosed but quite advanced cancer patients. She and her colleagues studied whether psychosocial factors — such as marital status, satisfaction with life, and hopelessness — bear any relationship to how long each patient lived or stayed in remission. Three years later she and her colleagues found no significant correlations. According to Dr. Cassileth, once the disease process is under way "it is the biology of the disease, and not psychosocial factors, that contributes to medical outcome."

If you believe the sick can make themselves well and your spouse doesn't believe it, will you accuse your spouse — inwardly or outwardly — of not trying? Is that accusation going to make you feel guilty? Or responsible for the sickness, because you couldn't make your regimen prevail? How responsible are we for our sicknesses? No one really knows.

Dr. Jimmie Holland, chief of psychiatry service at the Memorial Sloan-Kettering Cancer Center, wrote a letter to the *New York Times* a while ago in which she said that "while the study of links between emotions and hormonal and immune functions is challenging, it is premature to extrapolate early findings to patients being treated for cancer today." She went on to point out that patients seem to be blamed for not trying hard enough and that this follows the well-known ideology of blaming the victim when no more acceptable explanation can be found. "This," said Dr. Holland, "imposes an even greater burden on cancer patients and on their families by giving the impression that bad attitudes are responsible for their diseases." She received lots of mail from well spouses.

Dr. Holland said in a phone interview that "some notes said things like 'I felt so bad. I thought his illness was my fault.' There's a hype in our culture right now and a need to believe in mind over matter. It's probably good to feel responsible for your health up to a certain point. But after that point, you can't control everything. The surviving spouse should not feel responsible."

Let's talk with a psychiatrist who is also a practicing physician. Dr. Peter Knapp heads the Department of Psychosomatic Medicine at Boston University's Medical School. A dignified and sympathetic Dr. Knapp sits in his cheerful office in Boston, with its many comfortable chairs and a colorful abstract painting done by his wife. He sums up his version of mind over matter.

"There's a theory that's enunciated piously most everywhere

but not always taken so seriously — the theory that disease is multidetermined and multicausal. Some people are vulnerable to disease for psychosocial reasons. There is the genetic element and there are family patterns of behavior. In some families there's a tendency to somatize instead of blowing up, a tendency to keep things inside. This can show itself in a psychological way as depression. Or in a physical way as bodily disease. And then, of course, any given bodily disease may affect one part or another part of the body. There's yet another element, one's individual history. If there are psychological factors in the auto-immune illnesses, they go back to very early phases in life. A small segment of the personality gets sealed off, a segment of the self that brings conflict. It festers.

"We don't know what causal role such conflicts may play in the auto-immune illnesses, but we do see that their resolution often does seem to result in remission. For instance, a lupus patient improves after resolving lifelong conflicts by working through a difficult childhood in psychotherapy. I have no idea, for certain, what part of the improvement comes from psychotherapy.

"So that adds another dimension to any auto-immune disease. That makes it harder. Has the patient got his finger on the trigger of turmoil? The patient feels blamed, and those around him feel outraged about the blame and yet in their own hearts they sometimes find themselves blaming the patient, too. The spouse's own ambivalence gets stirred up.

"Being a good spouse to someone with a chronic illness is like being a good therapist or a good parent. One does as one does with a child, without being patronizing. You recognize, but you don't get enmeshed. You don't gratify every need or whim, just the most grown-up parts. It's extremely important that the spouse have some kind of life apart."

It's complex. It's ambiguous. You do the best you can. You don't get into a power struggle over it. You work on yourself, not your spouse. Colman and Krista handle lupus with a wise practicality. In their mid-thirties, they've lived six years now with Krista's lupus. This form of arthritis opens with an acute episode and moves, as Krista's has, to a latent or "time-bomb" phase. This may be followed by a another acute period and, perhaps, death. Krista reduces demands on herself as much as the mother of two young children can. She juggles: to simplify things, she abandoned her dream of a career, yet this very act adds the stress of disappointment. What about Colman? How does he handle the subtleties of what's called a stress-related illness?

I don't feel I have to walk on eggs or anything to avoid Krista's having stress. I feel I ought to, but I don't. I tend to be fairly immediate and intuitive. This is my management style, and when I'm managing people at work I get it right about 90 percent of the time. At home, it's harder.

It's more the second order effect that gets to you in the stress-related element. If Krista is having a flare-up, will that cause us a problem? Not the other way around. Will we have to cancel going out somewhere? Will I have to duck out from work and come home? If that happens, I feel bad and think, "Damn, this had to happen today!" But when I get an immediate kick-in of "How can I feel that way? Krista's not making this up! This is a real crisis. I shouldn't feel resentment." But it's tricky. It's only human to feel disappointment. The dividing line between disappointment and resentment is fairly small.

Pressures other than how stress affects Krista and the family loom much larger. And that is the basic message: the illness is a force that changes lives. Colman now works six and a half days a week designing computers and comes home Sunday noon to "spend the weekend" with the family.

Krista doesn't want to put pressure on me, but she feels the family needs are getting overrun by my work. We have pretty much reached the point where my income is completely adequate for the lifestyle we had originally expected with two incomes. How much is because I am prepared to work the kinds of hours and put in the energy I do? The joke around the house is that the money my employer pays me is the bribe I pay the rest of the family to let me go and have fun at work. I love the job I do. It's like playing, at last. Do I feel good that the illness lets me play more? I feel guilty. I feel it's really unfair that I get the benefit of Krista's misfortune. If she weren't sick, she would have a career and we would be doing the balancing act of two careers plus children. I would be home more.

The reduced energy of illness has far more effect on the life of this family than do the subtleties of stress. The changed work load and the split time cause some tension and asymmetry — and some isolation from each other. Here is Colman's day:

I fix the school lunches and one for myself. Some days I leave at 5:30 A.M. to get into the city before the rush hour, and I call Krista at 6:30. What time I get home varies. Krista probably cooks supper between half and two-thirds of the time. I cook the rest. On weekends I cook. She tends to flop. I really enjoy cooking.

I spend a fair amount of time with the kids. As much as other fathers, maybe. I don't go out drinking with the lads or off to sporting events. I am at home with the children evenings. By and large I try and give them as much attention as I can.

Krista goes to bed really early. I can function on five hours' sleep. We spend a little bit of time together in the evening and then she's off to bed and fast asleep. I'm still up. This causes a mismatch that causes us to be a little further apart. We don't discuss things as we are settling to sleep the way we used to. And there are decisions you make first thing in the morning, things to do with the kids: a child's crisis, "I've forgotten this" or "I'm sick." We don't handle those together.

When will the time-bomb phase give way to greater sickness? Waiting for this is itself a stress.

I went through a fairly stressed-out period back about three years ago. I felt up against it. What would I do if she dies? What would happen to the kids? It pops into my mind less and less. There's no firm data on expected life span with lupus. It can go into remission. Krista's has not gone into remission, but it has plateaued. It can flip at any time. I imagine she isn't going to change for the better. That she'll have minor flare-ups and maybe eventually one big flare-up. When it happens, I'll handle it. You second-guess or plan ahead so long and then you can't anymore. You adapt. It's like being in a different country driving on the other side of the road.

So save your time and money and what's left of your hope. Follow Angela's advice and stick with doctors you trust. We can't control everything. If we could, who would die? And if there were no illness, how would nature shed the old generation for the new? Do what you can for moderate diet and exercise. But don't fight. Don't get into controversy over the brown rice or the ice cream. Accept your spouse's view of how to treat the illness. It's easier. For long-term preventive medicine, the gurus may be right — but so far they can't walk into the cancer ward and cure half the patients.

Swat those mosquitoes.

# Chapter 11
# Biting the Dust

Money. It's green and crisp. It's silver and heavy. It's an abstraction that's shared by hundreds of screaming traders on Wall Street at the Exchange. I've always juggled it, paid half my college expenses, fed and bused and clothed myself at fifteen dollars a week through graduate school, saved a few thousand before the children came. My father said I was good with money. Everyone says if you work hard, you get it.

What innocence.

I was working harder than anyone I knew. Except maybe Jane.

I needed money for the children!

Time? You need time to get money. If you don't have enough of either one and less and less of both, watch out for the ground. You may be so downwardly mobile you bite the dust. For the next few years, I thought about little but money. It might perhaps have been easier if we were dirt poor (I doubt it) because then the edges of our economy wouldn't have been so blurred. We had occasional cleaning help, after all; we had a lovely old house, a rattling car.

Whatever the middle class is, the kids must stay in it. I argued this on Tuesdays and Fridays, and Ted argued it on Mondays and Wednesdays. On the third day of the month, I carried the government's check to the bank teller, feeling both grateful and ashamed. By middle class, we didn't mean color TVs; we didn't mean vacations; we did mean an occasional movie and a shot at college. Our families offered infusions of money, and sometimes we had to take it. "If you can't pay it back, consider it yours," they would say, making the loans both less than and more than a business deal. Borrowing made us feel small, failed. It made the lenders worry: Is this the beginning of financial dependency?

And it surely would have been easier if we weren't in the free-lance market. You never know what's happening there. Ted's life and times of Pericles might sell to a publisher and it might not. I could give up writing — the object of twenty years' effort — and take a low-paying job. Could I survive the resulting depression?

The first ad said you needed your own car and that the bar was in a remote location. The good part was the "high pay" for only two nights a week. I'd waited tables at college. I called from the five-and-ten.

"I'm calling about the job you advertised in the paper."

"Oh, yeah, what job?"

"The one for a waitress and barmaid two nights a week."

"Yeah?"

"What nights do you have in mind?"

"That depends, lady."

"How high is the high pay?"

"Come on, lady. First of all, how old are you?"

"I'm old enough. What's the age requirement?"

"Oh, come on, lady. You're the one looking for a job. If you think you can . . ."

I hung up and tried the next one. The canaries sang in their cages.

"How much does your night job of pin chaser pay?"

"Minimum, about twenty-seven a night."

"What exactly does a pin chaser do?"

That time, he hung up.

Substitute teaching paid thirty a day, but you needed degrees and certifications. All I had was a former national grant, a stack of published witticism, a B.A. and an M.A., an independent work history, a strong discipline, lots of energy for work, and a class advantage — which was rapidly being outweighed by an age disadvantage.

While they read my résumé at the nursing home where I'd applied for social director, I watched an old man with sad, obedient eyes walking to the water fountain and two women proceeding slowly with walkers. I viewed them differently now that Ted used a cane. The halls smelled of the fungi of waiting. How about a farm with rocking chairs and steaming stews and dogs and cats? With young people and students and babies? Unrealistic. I'd never get the job.

"I'm sorry," the young black-haired man said. "We can't even interview you. You are overqualified by life experience and underqualified in social directing."

The plants dried in the heat of my radiator. Gray slush covered Highfield's main street. Seth had finished eighth grade at the junior high and begun walking through town to the high school where he kept on as a Bookie, making friends and traveling with a small group of D & D-ers. He seemed happier. If I made a list of household chores, I could count on Seth to do his, nothing extra, but his allotment and on time. He cooked one night a week and could put a complete beef stew on the table at six. Debbie had finished sixth grade. The old junior high complex visible from my office window had been phased out and she bused to the town's single junior high —over-crowded and filled with low-morale teachers. If I dropped a handful of forks on the floor, Debbie would be there to pick them up. But she had trouble getting a salad on the table to go with the pizza she liked to warm up, and her marks kept slipping.

When you're downwardly mobile, you don't tend to a lot of the fine points. When you're a well spouse, life goes by almost as if you weren't living it. You don't get to the good things. You don't volunteer for the town library or take a casserole to a friend who broke an ankle or get up a really good birthday party. When you are forty-eight, men (well, most of them) stop looking at you on the street and you don't look at them either because you think of only one thing: money. That's why the plants were dry.

I filled the old milk bottle and watered them. I'd finished a sixty-page outline for somebody else's book on missing people. I'd drafted half a book for somebody else on sleep and dreaming. I'd taught two summer courses in editing. And I'd borrowed money from friends and family to launch an abortive book project of my own.

Okay. Okay.

Let's not get maudlin. Let's not feel sorry for ourselves.

Out on the street people walked gingerly through puddles. You're not the only one with troubles, kid.

Start over. Think in longer terms. The shortsighted planning of the desperate only assures that they'll never get a hold on the future. Item 1: Must stick with free-lance out of Manhattan because that's where your contacts and experience lie and because you can't find comparable pay in Highfield — the local paper offers writers fifteen dollars per feature article. Item 2: Get out of editing. It pays poorly. Item 3: Get out of ghostwriting. It pays well, but you can't multiply the product. You can't build on your own successes. Item 4: Forget humor, it's too chancy. Item 5: Try the magazine market. Launch a concerted attack.

Are you kidding? That classically impossible market?

Okay. Think.

Try the service end of magazines — steadier, more reliable. It'll still be tough. It'll take another year. By the time you're forty-nine, you may have some control over your livelihood. Advantage: writing your own stuff allows you to multiply. One good article can grow. Disadvantage: you go crazy. A quarter of the time you get kill fees instead of pay. Half the time you get nothing.

Okay. Okay.

Take a break now.

I stood up and ripped my new jeans on a nail in my desk chair.

"Oh, fuck it!" I shouted. "I quit!"


Mother Teresa, she's too far off. Besides, I could never raise the cash for a ticket to Calcutta. I called a psychotherapist.

"Ten sessions, that's absolutely all. When Blue Cross stops, I stop."

"What if you need more?" Dr. Feldman sounded reasonable.

"It's because of money that I'm going crazy. Besides, I spent far too many years with an earlier therapist. I need to know that I can get out."

He took me.

What a lovely man. Dr. Feldman would get tears in his eyes

when I got tears in mine. Something Ted couldn't do anymore.

"I live in a box," I began in his office, which was also filled with hanging plants, only his looked green and shiny. "And it's too small for me. At the right is a wall called Anxiety that I can't get over. When the mortgage is due and I don't have it, I live near that wall. Only I can't call it the mortgage money because Ted's disability pays the mortgage. He's always telling people that his disability covers food and shelter, Maggie pays for the incidentals. He has to say that for his self-esteem because he suffers over it. At the left of the box is a wall called Depression. When I can pay the mortgage, I live over there. In a sort of a heap like Debbie's puppy. I get to thinking that if I can pay the mortgage, why can't I climb out and do what I want?"

Dr. Feldman didn't tell me to hire a handyman.

"Where does it hurt?" Dr. Feldman told me to point to where it hurt. "Behind your eyes? In your throat? In your chest?"

Well, it was wonderful. I existed.

Dr. Feldman allowed me to spread the therapy out, once every three weeks over thirty weeks. He said I was skipping over my emotions too fast, not stopping to feel them. I was rushing to act, to remedy. Of course, I couldn't write. I was too preoccupied. Feeling the emotions would help. I should stop working whenever I felt sad and just feel sad.

"How does it feel?" Dr. Feldman asked over and over. He didn't give up, forget or fail to notice any hesitation or silence in those eight months during which we met. Emotions tell us what's good for us to do, he explained over and over. They help us make out our agendas for action more wisely. If I shoveled my emotions under the rug, no wonder I felt both frantic and paralyzed.

Ted's months of Imuran killed off some white cells and latent viruses surfaced. His ear began to ache all the time. He was even more tired. He quit the Historical Association because to attend their meetings one evening meant losing the next day's work time to fatigue. His right foot swelled up and turned red; it looked dead. Like an old man, he shuffled across the winter's ice. To keep him from getting isolated, I invited people to dinner. Visitors sitting on my mother's Persian rugs never guessed how financially desperate I felt. A third of our plans got canceled because Ted was too tired or because guests or hosts turned out to be contagious with flu or colds. There were nights I served a labor-intensive coq au vin to a grateful Ted and two resistant kids. After Christmas Ted's neurologist advised him to go off Imuran to build back his white cells: it wasn't doing any measurable good.

Ted simply would not entertain dark emotions, not from himself and (perhaps, therefore) not from anyone else. If the sick can't give voice to the pain, their well can't. And if you can't voice the pain, you can't feel any emotions.

"I'm not being overly pessimistic, for Pete's sake! There's no money. We're overdrawn four hundred and seventy dollars at the bank." I sat up in the bed in the brown-papered bedroom: we seemed to fight here most often.

"I had to get my tooth fixed!"

"Of course you did. That's the point. There's always something. The problem is larger. We need more money. I was just telling you how I felt. You don't have to do anything about it. I feel scared. That's all. I wanted you to know how I felt."

"You're always scared. We can borrow from Susan."

Resigned, Dr. Feldman, that's how I feel. I began talking to him in my head, as I lay nightly by the low window watching the maples against the street light. Resigned to the fact that I can't tell Ted about it.

My mother was in the hospital again, a slow kidney failure diagnosed. Seth asked for a pair of pants without holes.

"Damn it!" Outside Seth was cursing as he brought in the garage pails during a sleetstorm.

"Can you drill me in science?" Debbie had loved science as a child. In seventh grade she was doing poorly.

"When I finish the bills."

"What's wrong?" Ted would ask me once in a while when I was silent too long.

"I'm scared. I'm depressed."

"No, you're not. You're just tired."

Actually, you bastard, I am scared! You want to know where it hurts? In the back of the throat. And I am sad. You want to know where it hurts? In the belly. I want to throw up. Thank you, Dr. Feldman, I know I'm here. It helps.

Ted never wanted to know where it hurt.

He hurt more.

"Could you help Debbie with her drill while I finish the bills?"

"Just for a few minutes. I'm going up to bed."

Ted took Debbie's puppy (a cuddly thing to help with her falling spirits) walking and fell over the leash. He got inside the house and fell in the hall. He got up to bed. Seth stayed late at school practicing for the debate club. Debbie stayed the afternoon next door at her friend's. Most of Debbie's friends seemed to come from broken homes. One day when I got home I found a husband in pain, a yapping dog, a note saying we needed a $750 oil burner immediately, and a clothes washer that had finally broken, unfixably. There would never be more time than this, so I put on the taco stuffing to warm, drove to the nearest appliance store, bought a washer they'd install, drove back, and stuffed the tacos. Half an hour later we were at the emergency room discovering Ted had cracked his clavicle. Jane or another single parent might have squeezed in a few minutes to play Hearts before the kids went to bed. I spent those minutes looking for a drugstore open late to fill Ted's prescription.

Where was the family? Were the kids spending the day away from home or alone in their rooms because they were teenagers? Or were they escaping the gloom of the house? There wasn't time to figure it out. Where does it hurt? The whole house hurts, the couch cushions are swollen with pain, the rugs flat with despair.

At breakfast the next morning, I was buttering an English muffin when Seth began to sing as he laid out his corned beef with mustard on a grinder roll. *"Pardon me, Roy."* He sang as he cut the scallion neatly against the tabletop. *"Is that the cat that chewed the new shoes?"* We ad-libbed on through the rest of the "Chattanooga Choo Choo."

It feels good! Good!

As Ted worsened, he grew sadder. Four years is too much. No treatment left to hope over and the gates began breaking. The truth grew larger and darker every day, and more crushing.

"I don't know what to do." He began to talk one evening when it got warm enough to open the porch and sit in the fading glow of forsythia. "There is an island of silence inside of me."

"Say more. Tell me more. How does it feel?"

"There is no more."

"How about going to see Dr. Feldman? He's terrific."

"No more therapy."

I dreamt I was biking and I looked down and saw that the back tire was entirely flat and hanging off the wheel, coming apart, it could not be repaired.

"He's getting more depressed now," I told Dr. Feldman, sitting in his soft chair near the tissue box. "It's really so sad. He has such a good eye for architecture. He used to love to walk around New York looking at the façades of buildings. The other day we were making our way up to my office and I asked him to tell me how he saw the façades of Highfield, the way he used to in New York. He said he couldn't. He couldn't look up at them. He couldn't talk while he was walking. He needed all his energy to walk. He had to look at the sidewalk. It's so sad. What a waste! Ted's eyes are scratchy in the corner. That might mean he's going blind again. I found another seven-hundred-and-fifty dollar error in the books. We'll have to borrow another thousand from Susan or our parents. My mother is going into the hospital this week and I'll be going down to New Haven to help her. Yesterday I passed a cemetery in the car and a little voice said, 'Gee, that looks peaceful, just lying around.' Don't worry, I'm not the suicidal type. I can't discuss it with Ted. I can't say I'm terrified. That I'm mad I have to do everything. I can't say that. And I can't say it's kind of exciting, either. That I'd be proud if I could pull it off, support a family. No, I can't say that to Ted. It would kill him. So I'm saying it to you. And I know you want me to sit here and cry, but I can't because I'm too scared. When you're anxious, you don't cry. So I'll tell you where it hurts. It hurts in my throat, here, in my throat. I want to scream. And I don't want to scream. You know, sometimes it's hard for me to talk to you because, nice as you are, kind as you are, you're going home this evening to a wife who not only makes professional bucks but who will also have supper on the table for you and no matter how much I tell you, that won't change."

I didn't mention that they might make love.

On Debbie's thirteenth birthday, Ted was in the hospital for intravenous ACTH to prevent further degeneration in his right leg. The physiotherapy department prescribed a brace.

"I won't have the black leather shoe," he whispered to me in the gray ward full of old, sick men. "The Tiny Tim shoe. I won't have it."

God. Shit. Divinities and excrement, why are these two our swear words? Say something to Ted. What? What?

"I'm sorry, Ted. I'm sorry you have to wear a brace."

Tears started out from under his eyes. I lay on the bed next to him.

One Monday my weekly check for food and a trip to New York brought the balance to $8.31. The disability check wouldn't come for two more weeks. We needed food money by Monday. That night I set the alarm for 7 A.M. and lay there planning Tuesday. I'd work six hours in my office and then head to the city. In person, I might be able to persuade old friends, old editors to give me quick work — work that didn't need a proposal or a speculative draft. Then I'd pick up Debbie at Jane's where she'd gone after spending a week with a friend in the city and we'd check in at her eye surgeon's and oh, yes, don't forget to load the raveling rug into the car to drop at the repair shop. Deep in the night I woke to the crash I'd been subliminally dreading for years. It seemed nearby, very near.

"Ted? Are you all right?"

His voice was strange, muffled.

"What? What?" I got the light on. He was sitting in a heap on the floor by the bed with his hand over his nose and mouth and there was blood all over his pajamas, his hand, the floor.

"I hurt my nose." Voice muffled by fingers.

"Take your hand away, Ted, oh Teddie."

There was a wide cut on his nose, the kind where you take the kids for stitches. He'd gotten up to go to the bathroom and lost his balance, striking his nose on the opened drawer of the night table as he fell.

"I'll get ice." Our kids had never needed stitches, only ice. I ran downstairs and shoved some ice cubes into a plastic bag and picked up the kitchen phone.

"Of course we're open," the man replied. "That's what an emergency room is for!"

So I wasn't functioning too well. I ran upstairs and saw Ted standing in the bathroom looking into the mirror under the harsh light of the bare bulb.

"It's stopped bleeding." He spoke in a slow, mechanical way. "But I'm going to be disfigured. My face will look different. It won't be me."

"We're going for stitches."

"I think I'd rather rest." He kept peering into the mirror.

"We have to go for stitches!"

"I'm too tired for that." He turned and began dragging his right foot back to the bed. He sat on the edge of it, looking very white. I set the ice on the bed.

"Aren't you going to get dressed?"

"I can't move." He looked so frozen, thin, skeletal, paralyzed. "I'm too . . . tired. I'll rest first."

Do something, Maggie!

"They're waiting for us at the emergency room. Come on, I'll help you get dressed."

It took twenty minutes for us to get Ted's clothes on. He'd never let me help him dress before. His right foot felt like a log or stone going into the sneaker. I left a note for Seth. Together we made our way down the porch stairs through the spring dark to the car.

In the narrow room, the surgeon placed an enormous green cloth over Ted's body. His nose stuck through a small circle cut into the cloth. The surgeon threaded the needle. He stitched.

"You were in shock," the surgeon explained to Ted. He placed an ordinary Band-Aid over the stitches. He handed me the list of what to watch out for in the next few days, mostly infection.

Shock?

Remember that.

I handed Ted his cane and gave him my arm: "This way to the limo, monsieur." We walked silently and slowly into the daybreak illuminating the parking lot.

Jane was expecting me for a late supper in Manhattan. Debbie's famous eye surgeon would shut the busy pages of his calendar book and not give us another appointment until fall: her eyes seemed worse. But should I go?

"Go," Ted said, in the driveway. "I'll be fine." I parked

under the maple, caught a glimpse of the fir trees that rose over the garage in their mysterious morning stillness, and walked around to open the door for Ted.

We got up onto the porch and into the dining room.

"Coffee and a bagel, thanks." He sat.

I threw away the note for Seth, made breakfast, and brought it to the round table. Sunrise outside, smell of coffee. Upstairs, a faint ringing. My alarm clock.

At four that afternoon I walked home from my office to see Ted, who insisted he was fine. Seth helped me load the nine-by-twelve rug into the car. I hugged him goodbye, not saying, "Take care of Daddy." It looked as if Seth needed a little care himself. At quarter of five, I turned off the highway, but no roads led to where I remembered the rug repair shop to be. All roads led to weedy vacant lots or bridges over urban decay, places where girls were raped or hid their aborted babies. My voice broke over the phone as I begged the storekeeper to stay open a few minutes more while I found my way to him. I couldn't park a car with even a battered old Persian rug in it overnight in Manhattan, and I couldn't afford to garage the car: I had no viable options.

You're just a little ragged, I told myself when I left the rug store. I pulled off the highway again for supper at six and found a suburban complex that contained a dance studio and a pizza parlor. Three dollars would have to do it for this meal. I ordered mushrooms on my slice and watched the couples in the dance studio learning *one two three la conga* — steps that could be employed nowhere anymore but in the ballrooms of ocean liners making luxury passage to sunlit beaches. *Café, madame? Voulez vous le chocolat ou l'orange?* Handsome strangers, croissants on silver trays, ball gowns of crepe du chine, myself a young woman with a future. Suddenly remembering (exactly how much?) the toll booths of Sputen Dyvel, I canceled my Coke and took ever smaller bites of my slice.

"You look awful," Jane said, opening the multilocked door of her brownstone apartment. "What's the matter?"

"Ted fell down. He was in shock. I couldn't find the rug store. I mixed up the Cross County with the Cross Bronx."

Debbie looked up from the floor where she sat watching TV with Patrick.

"It's okay, honey, Daddy's okay." I walked toward the kids.

"Sit down," Jane said. "I'll make you some tea."

When she handed me the tea, a great lump came into my throat. Later, in the privacy of the kitchen, I told her about the crash, the disorientation, the blood, the needle through the skin, the scar — I'll look in the mirror and it won't be me. Our lives were like that. We weren't ourselves anymore.

"You know what I do?" I went on, unable to stop talking. "I come home every day and read 'Your Stars Today' in the newspaper. I've discovered why the poor and oppressed read that stuff. It's the only place you can get a sixty-forty success rate, which is a hell of a lot better than I'm doing in the magazine market."

Jane took over. "Sit right there. I'm bringing you some ham. Even if you're not hungry. You need somebody to bring you something."

I sat.

"Now promise me this." She handed me the plate. "You will never, ever take over the physical nursing, if it comes to that."

Debbie hadn't even told me her week in New York. Or if she had, I hadn't even heard it.

One editor told me at a sixty-seven-dollar lunch that he hadn't immediate work, maybe in October. So it went, all day. Wednesday night I didn't sleep. At least there was the appointment I had at home Friday night to interview an economist visiting a nearby college. *Savvy* wanted a piece on that. It was the only solid money in sight.

At Debbie's eye appointment, her surgeon assured me there was no problem. She was developing a near eye and a far eye, like Ted's. True, her eyes were less parallel, but that was simply a cosmetic problem. If it bothered her in a couple of years, we could consider a third surgery. I gave her a dollar to buy a yogurt for lunch off a street cart and went on to a business lunch: veal in wine, white linen, and a sprig of roses. The editor said no work, but maybe I'd like to limn out a proposal for a piece on adolescents and music, pure speculation. I'd have to pay for my own phone calls for the interviews. Hard science, he wanted, facts, studies. I picked up Debbie outside the Museum of Modern Art and we headed north. She wore the Sony Walkman that Jane had given her as a late birthday present. Sid and Mim had provided some tapes.

"Andy has his own stereo," Debbie said, as I avoided the potholes on the Cross Bronx.

"Jane took Patrick and me out to dinner twice," she reported near Stamford. "Once to Chinese and once to Japanese."

Could I hate my own daughter?

Near Bridgeport, it started to rain.

"You know," — Debbie took one earmuff off one ear — "I never did understand how raindrops know where to end themselves."

I loved her!

"Or," she added, as she replaced the earmuff and shouted at me against the noise of her own internal state, "how the universe stops wherever it stops, either."

"What a beautiful . . ."

She was gone, tuned out. Why was she getting C's in science? No. No. No. No more problems. Time to relax. It's Seth's night to cook. He's a good cook. God, I'm tired. It's something to look forward to. This is time to enjoy. It's not time to worry. A couple of hours' peace on the highway. Ted's fall is finished. Ted's okay. Just a couple of hours' peace and then you can deal with the economic disaster of New York. Work Saturday. Work Sunday. Turn in the economist interview. Use up all the canned and frozen foods. They'll last a week.

The house seemed strangely quiet.

"I have a fever." Ted lay in bed. The surgeon's Band-Aid was still on his nose. His forehead felt hot. I got the thermometer.

"Where's Seth?"

"In bed. Sore throat."

Ted: 101. Seth: 102.

"Grape juice." Seth lay in the blue room too exhausted to read. There was a big white lump on his tonsils.

"You'd better change my bandage now. I couldn't get it off." I sat on our bed and pulled hesitantly at the patch of gauze on Ted's nose. When it came up, the skin began to come with it, pulling at the black thread of the stitches, making it ooze blood and a pink pus.

"Hi, Dad." Debbie stood at the door. "Are you okay?"

"Had a little fall but I'm fine. How was New York?"

"I got a Sony Walkman. When do we eat?"

When she left, Ted said he thought he had blood poisoning. I got out the surgeon's instruction sheet.

"Looks like what they describe as infected. I'll call the hospital to find out how to get this bandage off."

A nurse said the surgeon was crazy to put on an ordinary Band-Aid. Soak it in peroxide.

It peeled right off.

"Looks a little red, the paper mentions red. It's infected. I shouldn't have gone to New York."

The emergency room was pretty crowded. A doctor put some salve on Ted's nose. Otherwise, fine. Fever from the infection, infection from the stitches.

"I'm going to ask him to look at my foot," Ted told me as he sat in the hospital wheelchair.

"What for?" I bent over and put my arm on his shoulder, thin. How was Seth? Was he awake. Had Debbie taken him more grape juice?

"Remember? I told you I had a splinter."

Oh, yes. He'd mentioned a splinter just as Seth and I were rolling up the rug on Tuesday.

"Maybe that's what's infected, not my nose. Maybe that's why I have the fever."

"Oh, come on! It says right in the sheet the surgeon gave me that you can get infections from the stitches. The doctor here just said that was it. Let's get home."

Seth needed me.

And I was totally exhausted.

In the morning as I was getting dressed, Ted asked me to look at the sole of his left foot.

I tucked in my shirt and moved to the foot of the bed. I dug out the sheet and stooped down to his foot.

"My God." It was practically green, the whole ball of his foot. Beyond ice. Beyond peroxide.

"Can you call the surgeon yourself? Get an appointment around four o'clock. That'll give me time to draft a memo on music and get my questions ready for the economist I have to see at six. I'll pick you up at quarter of four."

Seth was still hot. He was trying to read through smudged glasses. I left his juice and crackers. His legs came so far down in the bed. When had he been growing? There was no time to see his growing. He would turn fifteen in days. No presents. What to get? When to get them? I didn't even know what he would want anymore.

At the surgeon's I kept on working, scanning the pages of

*Travel and Leisure.* Would they want my old piece on Cyprus?

"You know anybody on *People?*"

"No." Ted sat with his left leg out on the magazine table.

When it was our turn, he leaned heavily on my arm. He couldn't put much weight on his good foot now.

"Blood poisoning," a new surgeon diagnosed abruptly, from the end of the examining table. "Gangrene. I'm going to cut it out. Don't move."

Ted winced.

"I told you not to move, Mr. Greenstein!"

"It's a leg tremor. I couldn't help it."

The surgeon moved to the middle of the table and showed us the red line.

"It's very faint," I said, guiltily, horrified.

"Gets up beyond the thigh and you've got permanent kidney damage. I'm putting him in for intravenous antibiotic."

At quarter of six I canceled my appointment with the economist. At quarter of seven I walked Seth into the emergency room for a throat culture.

Strep.

Sterilize everything. Ted mustn't get strep.

Ted came home using a walker. He refused to let me rent a wheelchair. He refused to move downstairs. He'd climb up the stairs on his backside, he would. And that's what he did. Oh, noble. Oh, heroic. I was supposed to cheer.

Is this it? Is he bedridden now?

Empty my urinal.

Bring me my juice.


Dr. Feldman suggested that I had never finished mourning my own father. This seemed ludicrous. My father had been dead for twenty years. Dr. Feldman told me to go visit his grave. His grave? I'd spent a summer reading my father's papers; I chatted with him in imagination at red lights, anytime. What did I need to visit his grave for? I went.

Two towns away from the cemetery, I felt warm tears rolling down my face. Great fructifying tears; I heard an inner voice finding the right word for Dr. Feldman from an old poem I'd read in graduate school. Tears like rain, fertile-making tears, unpainful. Where does it hurt? Why, it doesn't hurt at all! It feels terrific! Miles and miles of tears here behind the steering wheel. And then I was standing in the cemetery with all my tears about me, wrapped in them, and what I felt was the certainty of being enveloped by the love my father had had for me. *You are loved* came the sense, not exactly a voice, emanating from the grass and the small fir bushes and the pale, gray stones.

So I sat and cried and was loved.

# Chapter 12

# What to Watch Out for in Therapy and in Support Groups

Now we climb out of the swamp of the chronic emotions. We'll never climb way out, but some things do help. Therapy might. This panacea of our century isn't foolproof. Psychiatrists and therapists can be awful. They can be superficial and have absolutely no idea what you're dealing with. They can be people you wouldn't spend ten minutes with if you didn't have to. So why should you learn life wisdom from them? Because some of them can be splendid — intuitive, deeply warm, and constructively tough.

How do you find a good one? You shop around. Visit three therapists. Call first and say, "Dr. So and So, I want to make an appointment for a consultation to see if we would be able to work well together." You are the buyer. Don't let the power structure of the doctor-patient twosome overcome you before you even begin therapy. Money spent on consultations now will be money saved on sessions later. Avoid obvious incompetence. A psychiatric social worker stood up last winter and explained to a group of people that "a functionally impaired person is someone who . . . uh . . . has an impairment . . . in . . . uh . . . functioning."

"I have a nastly little acid test for therapists," one man confesses. "I skip anybody who hits the scales at more than forty pounds overweight, anybody who looks wooden, and anybody who speaks in jargon, including using 'right' or 'okay' after every sentence. But if a therapist can make me laugh," he admits, "he's okay, no matter what." This man is right. Laughing is the flip side of crying, and it means you'll be able to connect.

Do you need therapy? Consider it if you've become empty of feelings or so frightened you think of little but trouble and find nothing to enjoy. Talking to a therapist doesn't mean you're mentally or emotionally ill. It can mean you're in a tough spot and need someone to listen. Who else can you tell your angers and fears to? Not your spouse, not all your grubbiest feelings. Not your family, they'd worry too much or begin to advise you on what to do. Not your spouse's family, that would seem disloyal. And not your friends, you'd bore and alienate them. A therapist may be perfect.

What kind of therapist? The following list is designed to give an overview of what's available. Be advised that two hundred members of the American Psychiatric Association are laboring to put out an official manual of recommended treatments for mental and emotional disorders. Little agreement has emerged and the manual grows to encyclopedic length. "There are four hundred and sixty brand-name therapy techniques last time I counted," reports Dr. T. Byram Karasu, director of the Department of Psychiatry at the Bronx Municipal Hospital, and the man who is orchestrating the manual.

There is no science to psychiatry, it's still an art. Shop as long for a professional helper as you would for a used car. And if you do get a lemon, dump him.

### LONG-TERM INDIVIDUAL THERAPY

Classical Freudian psychoanalysis has slowly given way (although not entirely, of course) to an eclectic potpourri of "the talking cure" practiced by any number of psychiatrists, most of whom consider the people they treat patients rather than clients. Psychoanalytical psychotherapy demands that the patient examine his emotions in terms of his history and labor to reach buried emotions rising from forgotten episodes; the therapist may say little or nothing at all. Cognitive therapy involves a close look at daily thoughts and feelings: are our automatic responses or our customary self-reproaches valid? Would we manage better if we didn't always carry certain inaccurate conclusions in the back of our minds? Behavioral therapy teaches relaxation techniques that still anxiety and allow us to function better or without panic in troubling situations.

### SHORT-TERM INDIVIDUAL THERAPY

Short-term therapy consists of ten or twelve sessions developed partly out of clients' need to "get finished" before their insurance coverage runs out. Since time is short, focus may be on one or two agreed-upon issues. The well spouse can simply say, "I'm scared and mad and bored and I want someone to hold my hand and tell me I'm terrific once a week for ten weeks." The therapist won't do either of those things, but he or she will corroborate that you're in a tough spot and will steer you around to what's actually happening if your own sense of reality has gotten skewed.

### COUPLES THERAPY

The therapist serves as a third party whose presence may help liquefy unexpressed resentments between you and your spouse. It won't change the basic situation (he's sick; she's sick) but it may open up awareness. Seek a therapist who won't be primarily compelled by the drama of sickness. You might even ask if the therapist has lived with sickness in his own family.

### SEX THERAPY

This provides a structured system of retraining in physical contact. Be sure to check for physical causes of sexual dysfunctioning first.

### FAMILY THERAPY

A generation of American therapists since the 1950s has developed what's called systems or family therapy, a way of dealing with individuals by monitoring relationships within the entire network of the family. Individuals are seen and taught to see themselves as members of twosomes and threesomes within a larger interrelating system and to examine what roles they play there and what roles are cast upon them by others. Personal history grows to include the history of your own and your spouse's parents, as the system extends backward a generation. It also extends forward to your children's experience.

Watch for this: does your therapist assume pathological behavior on your family's part? Or does he or she truly grasp the reality of the practical and emotional stress of chronic (not acute) illness?

## GROUP THERAPY

Here patients or participants learn not from the latter-day nurture of an artificial "parent" as in the doctor-patient twosome, but through exposure to artificial siblings. Such groups may be offered by psychiatrists in conjunction with individual long-term therapy, or they may be offered alone on a long- or short-term basis.

If you're severely depressed (not hungry, can't sleep, no point in living), you may want medication. For prescriptions, you need a psychiatrist with an M.D. degree. A clinical psychologist has spent four years in graduate school to acquire a Ph.D. and is not licensed to prescribe drugs; they tend to want to give batteries of tests. A psychiatric social worker has spent two years in graduate school in a master's program for an M.S.W. degree. This may be a good bet for the well spouse. The lower down the training ladder you go, the less dogma attaches itself to the therapy. Psychiatric social workers may be enormously practical and supportive, which is apt to be exactly what the well spouse craves. Less orthodox and more eclectic, Jungian therapists offer a combination of mothering, mythic personality typing, and self-improvement that could both distract and nurture the well spouse.

In therapy, watch out for this danger: don't accept a therapist's suggestion that you look deep into past history unless it's really relevant. Deal with situational pain before you put years into reconstructing your whole personality. And this: don't sit passively by in family or couples therapy while all the attention goes to children or the sick spouse. Voice your sense of oppressive responsibility.

Maybe you don't need knowledgeable therapists but knowledgeable fellow travelers, people who have walked in your own moccasins. That's the second option: try a support group. What kind?

Earlier in the century, Alcoholics Anonymous presented a successful model for support groups of all stripes and flavors. Now you find groups listed willy-nilly in local newspapers or posted on the bulletin boards of hospitals: Compassionate Friends for parents who have lost a child; Parents Without Partners; Grown Children of Alcoholics. Is there a group for us? The Weekly Well Spouses? Could we meet for lunch and talk and eat and laugh a little? Or to hike? No, not yet. (But see Appendix A, the final entry.)

Once in a great while, you can find a support group for the spouses of people with particular illnesses. These are run through the local chapters of the illness's national association. To find your chapter, contact the national headquarters of the illness in question (see Appendix A). Well spouses meeting with each other may be the best sort of group for you. Such a meeting is described in a personal way in chapter 19.

More frequently available groups are described in this chapter. The first two kinds can be helpful if you don't expect too much or the wrong thing from them. These information workshops and ongoing support groups focus rightly on the sick, not on the needs of the well spouses. Information workshops serve to educate the newly diagnosed and their partners in the management of a particular illness. They cover symptoms and causes, diet, exercise, use of special equipment, self-testing, management of medication, and common emotional problems. The pluses: you both learn lots of practical stuff; you realize you're not the only couple hit with this particular bad news. The minuses: the well spouse belongs on the periphery here and that's exactly the emotional location from which she may need relief. To find one, call your hospital or watch the local paper. Workshops tend to be one-nighters or to last three of four sessions. What are they like?

INFORMATION WORKSHOP: DIABETES TYPE II

How quiet the hospital conference room seems, how still. All but one of the five men and four women patients look overweight. The three well wives and a daughter sit more trimly beside them.

The young and warmly professional diabetes teaching nurse stands at the end of the table, explaining how Type II diabetes comes on. It happens slowly with symptoms of tiredness, itchiness, and blurry vision, or no symptoms at all. The body's blood sugar can't get into cells and runs off into the fluids of the eye or out via the urine. Simple overweight can bring on diabetes II (which used to be called "senile"), but when you're developing it, you may lose a lot of weight all of a sudden as the sugar runs off. If you have diabetes, you must try to lose weight. However, the illness itself — if not well controlled — makes you crave food, and so does the insulin you may or may not have to take.

The patients begin to respond. They nod. One describes how a five-mile ride on her stationary bike only makes her hungrier — causing her to root around in the pantry even harder.

The teaching nurse continues. A diabetic's routine of carefully measured, carefully timed feedings can make you feel confined.

"Amen," the patients attest to this.

Then there's fear. Diabetes can age and damage you. If blood sugar goes up, so does blood fat. The bigger arteries may clog, leading to stroke or heart attack. The smaller arteries may clog, damaging the tiny vessels of the retina and blinding you or filling the tiny arteries of the kidneys and making you dependent on dialysis. Nerves may process information askew: you might feel heat when there isn't any, or tingling, or pain. Nerves in the erectile tissue of the penis can scramble messages, too: one out of four male Type II diabetics may grow impotent.

The male patients make jokes.

The females remain silent.

Tiny clogged arteries in the feet can bring gangrene and amputation. But don't be afraid. Learn how to take care of yourself and chances are you can escape these frightening possibilities.

The well wives ask practical questions about diet. This is no place for them to bring up their fear.


DIET WORKSHOP: HEART PATIENTS

"Go on using your favorite recipes," the dietitian in her emerald green dress urges the three men and two women in the small classroom. "Just reduce the animal fats and salts and sugars, or eliminate them entirely, or substitute buttermilk and cornstarch for sour cream."

She shows slides of the enemy, fat marbled red meat. She explains polyunsaturated and monounsaturated and hydrogenized a second and a third time because "it's so confusing! I know it's confusing!"

At one slide, a quiet man asks, "Is that catsup in the bottle by the olives?"

"No," she says. "It's soy sauce, very salty. Don't worry, catsup is okay!"

The man looked relieved.

At how many meetings do patients listen to experts younger than themselves?

"That's tofu," the dietitian explains. "I can't get my own family to embrace it cheerfully, but it's terrific. No flavor of its own but no cholesterol, either." This beautiful young woman has a waistline and a husband and young children; she refers to her cakes and cookies in the present tense. She speaks to her patients from a lost era in their own lives.

"You're not the Tofutti generation," she quips. "I know how you feel. I'm not a health food nut myself." She labors not to patronize her listeners. But she patronizes at every turn, simply by having a waistline and bright hair.

Another young nurse wheels in the decaf, while the dietitian serves hommus with whole wheat pita from a basket she's decorated with freshly picked mint and basil and oregano.

The talkative patient (there's one in every group) sees the mint. "Mint julep!" he recalls exuberantly. "I remember one night in college, a friend was giving a party and he said, 'Hey, go into that garden and get some mint.' So we climbed over the wall and picked us some mint and made us the best drinks! We passed them around, saying 'Have some of this mint julep' — only it turned out to be catnip. That was some party!"

Everyone laughs.

The nurse and the dietitian exchange a quick look, their blue young eyes connect. They don't quite smile. Here's what I might have thought at thirty: *Can you believe these duffers?*

We over-fifties exchange our own look with our own blue old eyes. Our look has no words but is full of the great, sweet poignancy of middle and older age: we can imagine the hearts of the young but they can't know ours — not yet.

"I've got to go home now," the quiet man says after his hommus, "and get to bed early. So I can get up in the morning . . ." He pauses, and finally adds ". . . hopefully!"

Suddenly, everyone laughs in a common nervous burst.

I feel the fear lurking in those chests. This is no place for a well spouse to tell her loneliness: it pales to nothing beside life's basic anxiety.

Ongoing support groups for the sick and their partners give more than information and can run for years. These may be social groups with picnics and Christmas parties. Some, especially newer groups, favor organizing for advocacy. The program varies from lectures on rights or the newest research to display of special equipment and to psychological issues. The minuses: it takes more courage than either of you may have or want to have to see the late-stage effects of the illnesses. One or the other of you may bolt at the sight of wheelchairs or crutches or nose hoses. You also need (and here's a good place to develop it) the knack of mixing comfortably with strangers from different socioeconomic niches. And last, too much of a support group may seem like too much focus on the illness. The pluses: information, inspiration, and community — what more could you want, except a cure?

Chapter Meeting, Arthritis Foundation

What a lot of energy in this room! Tonight it's a round-robin. The chairperson begins by sayng she's had both rheumatoid knees operated on.

"They don't hurt anymore." She stands comfortably before the group. She keeps a job, loves her grandchildren, and misses her recently deceased husband.

A bubbly grandmother with fingers surgically reconstructed says she started out depressed. Her husband left and her oldest child couldn't deal with the illness. Once she decided to get on with life, she'd learned to live each day and enjoy: she paints, plays the piano, and sings in a choir.

A woman with no obvious symptoms of her painful fibrocitis and osteoarthritis recites her motto: "I do *what* I can, *when* I can, *if* I can, and the *best* I can."

An older woman ends her account with "But I beat that

problem and, with the grace of Almighty God, I'll beat this! Or keep going, anyway!"

Everyone applauds.

It feels like a pep rally. The well spouses cheer and applaud; they don't speak.

A shapely grandmother with one set of fingers awry and the other surgically realigned displays some nail clippers and shows how to elongate them with bits of wood to get more control. She demonstrates a jar opener with a leather thong. She raises up the Swiss army knife she carries at her belt for an extra digit. She copes, with great ingenuity.

Then a well family member speaks. She needs help. She can't get her mother out of bed.

"She's got to get up!"

"Ask the intern for a mood elevator."

Voices from all around offer suggestions; these veterans know what to do, they remember being depressed.

"Get the mental health office to send a psychiatric helper."

"Tell her all meals will be served at the table."

The advice is practical, expert.

"Make her bed up when she goes to the bathroom."

"She's got to get herself ready to fight!"

It's a very resourceful bunch. The well spouse, however, sits on the bench of this team. If he doesn't feel like cheering, he may begin to feel guilty.

CHAPTER MEETING, AMERICAN LUNG ASSOCIATION'S BETTER BREATHERS

"The standard problem with COPD is of not knowing," says the teaching nurse to the large group of men and women in the small auditorium on a lecture night. "Have you got asthma or bronchitis or emphysema? One trip the doctor says it's mostly bronchitis and on the next visit he says it's mostly asthma. You don't feel quite sure what you've got or how you should medicate. He gives you prednisone one time and changes the doses every day. The next time he tries a new drug."

She explains why this is typical of COPD and the questions move to the side effects of prednisone. She lists them in Magic Marker: damage to bones, swelling of face, buildup of hump behind neck, itching, false peppiness.

"Over the long haul, can't the cortisones kill you?" The question comes from the audience.

"Why don't you answer that?" The nurse calls on a patient familiar to her.

An active-looking gray-haired woman in a kelly green jacket stands up. "I guess I'd better take off my jacket for this, so you can see how bent I am." In a matter-of-fact way, she removes the jacket and pats a small hump below her neck. Little else looks unusual. She appears strong, capable. "I've been taking prednisone since nineteen fifty-nine," she says with an optimistic lilt. "And I'm still here. I'm working full-time. I have hobbies and friends. I bike and I travel. I have the hump. And here," she touches her chin, "I'm swollen so that my face isn't my own in the mirror. But I'm alive! I'm alive! So don't be afraid if you have to take prednisone." She puts on her jacket and sits down to applause.

A middle-aged woman speaks from the other side of the aisle. "I've been on prednisone for years. I have my good days and my bad. On my bad days I lie on my couch reading. On my good days, I ride a bike and cook. I take a walk. I hike. I can even have sex."

Whistles! Wild applause!

Who wouldn't be drawn in? Perhaps a well spouse who is very, very tired.

CHAPTER MEETING, I.A. AND I-ANON

Ten men, one woman, one male nurse, and one male doctor, one female psychologist: with fear and trembling does one approach the door. The atmosphere within relaxes and liberates. It's plain comfortable language spoken here with emphasis — at this particular meeting, anyway — on the latest (third generation) of flexile penile implant and on pharmacological erection therapy (PET; sometimes it's Program, or PEP). There are now 150,000 men walking the streets with implants. It's the last choice, however, considering the surgery and the expense — perhaps eight thousand dollars for the overnight job, if you don't have coverage. The chemical injections are much more affordable, working out to about the price of a pair of movie tickets per erection.

One man told how he'd become impotent without realizing it during the last years of his wife's illness. He wished to return to sexual intercourse after her death, and when the injection program didn't work for him, he took the implant. It changed his life. Now he's married again and engaging in intercourse frequently. He sounded very happy.

Another man spoke for the injections. His partner handled the tiny needle. Anticipation of what was to come outweighed the small pain. He, too, was deeply grateful for the return of erection.

A third and disgruntled man had found that neither an operation to correct leakage (of the trapped blood that stiffens the penis; blood can leak back through the veins into the body and this may be the most common cause of erectile dysfunction) nor the injection therapy had worked. He was considering the implant.

Then a young visitor spoke movingly. For several years he'd had trouble with erections. Doctors had told him it was in his head. He knew it wasn't. He just knew. But the doctors wouldn't listen! The therapists wouldn't listen! There were women he wanted to ask out, but he didn't even dare take a woman to dinner anymore, lest he get involved. But now that these men had spoken . . . he was impressed with how freely they spoke . . . now, maybe, there was hope.

This was a wonderful moment.

A couple would find that such meetings break through their isolation; a well spouse alone could see impotence as a group rather than personal phenomenon.

———◆———

## AND NOW A WORD FROM THE WOMEN . . .

*Injection Program,* New York wife: "He was very nerved up and it didn't seem to do. He got half an erection and that was it. It's going to destroy the marriage unless I learn to say to hell with it."

*Implant,* New Jersey wife: "Our troubles started after his whole body radiation and his year of chemotherapy. He'd have an erection for a minute and then ejaculate. I felt I was causing it. I got angry. He got angry. He fell into a huge depression. So did I. We got close to a divorce. They made us do therapy. Then he saw an article and went for a sleep test and found his problem was physiological. He decided on the implant. It was an option on the Medicare at my office. We're very happy with it! I keep feeling I might be wearing it out! It took us a while to get back together emotionally, but now we spend hours talking at night again. Both our depressions have lifted."

———◆———

Let's turn to a third kind of group, one more directly helpful to us — family support groups. In her Brooklyn house over the subway line, the sculptor Leah remarked that sickness brings as much emotional pain as physical, if not more. "Anybody with a chronic illness needs lots of psychological counseling and so do their families. As it is now, the psychological treatment is considered a luxury and the physical a necessity. But if you asked most people involved with chronic illness, they would reverse that order. You have to sort out the nasty feelings. Clarity is beyond price. It's the ultimate good."

In family support groups, lots of information gets passed around and lots of nasty feelings aired. Here at last the chronically well feel safe enough to express without guilt their frustration, disappointment, and anger. Or just their fear, their sorrow. You'll find less of the jollity that often marks the group for the sick. The sick do seem to evidence a sense of being onstage in their groups, of performing spiritedly for others. The well appear, at least initially, too tired. Unfortunately for those whose spouses are physically disabled, most groups cluster around illnesses that affect cerebral functioning.

NURSING HOME SUPPORT GROUP FOR FAMILY MEMBERS OF PEOPLE WITH ALZHEIMER'S

The only man in a business suit, a visiting lawyer tells this group of thirty men and women that you start proceedings to declare someone incompetent with a certificate from the doctor. With that, you petition a probate court. Timing is tricky. Long before anyone shows signs of incompetency ("You mean at the altar?" one woman interrupts), he or she should have signed certain papers: a Durable (not a General) Power of Attorney, for example, and proper ownership papers. Couples should hold property as "tenants in common" and not — as most of us do — jointly or as "tenants by entirety." Holding an asset in common means you can split it half and half when you need to. And you may need to if one of you has to be put in a nursing home.

"In other words, we should all learn all these things before we're out in left field!" another woman comments edgily.

"But how can you go out and learn them when someone trails you twenty-four hours a day?" another asks.

Three themes recur throughout the meeting: the need to know things ahead of time, the inexpressible difficulty of caring for someone with brain damage, and the ubiquitous family squabbling in such cases.

"The children don't see it. You have to live with it to believe it."

"Why are all the laws for the sick? Don't we count? We are the victims."

"Her sisters are fighting me. They don't want me to put her in because her name will be in the newspaper."

When the attorney leaves, the group leader moves skillfully out of information into the much-needed support.

Sometimes those present refer to their charges not by name but as "Mine", this way: "Mine burnt himself." "I put the Depends on mine and he pulls them off unless I put shorts on top."

"When we talk together, we find out we're not alone!" one woman says, as the mood begins to change.

"And we find out we're not very well informed!" Another calls out, laughing at last.


MEETING: FAMILY SURVIVAL PROJECT, SAN FRANCISCO

This group was formed in 1976 for the families of brain-damaged people, and this meeting takes place on a summer night in a YMCA basement room. Three attend: a middle-aged woman whose husband has Alzheimer's, a younger woman whose mother has it, and a still younger women whose husband's diagnosis is yet uncertain — although he's been on disability for a year and her doctor has referred her to this group.

The younger woman introduces herself and her situation. Her husband is forgetful, there have been personality changes. Yet even this morning new tests proved inconclusive. Lines of worry mark her handsome face. Her children are not yet in college. She fidgets with her paper napkin as she tells of her fear and frustration in trying to figure out what's what.

"You've got to keep going back and back and back." The gray-haired older wife leans forward and begins to tell her own tale. "It took me three years to get my husband's diagnosis. When it came I cried for days, weeks. And then I stopped crying." She explains how she hires a man by the hour to take her husband out to baseball games — games whose plays he forgets and whose scores he can't remember. "I've lost my companion," she adds poignantly. "My husband talked, always talked. We were both good talkers. We'd go out to a restaurant and talk through dinner. The rest of the married couples — some of them would just sit there, staring. They had nothing to say to each other anymore. We still had plenty to say, my husband and I. Now that's gone. It's as if he's dead. I have my husband. But he's not there." A particular jazz concert someone had taken her to brought her back into life. She'd found herself tapping her foot and singing.

"Me too!" The younger wife leans forward. "I went to that same concert!"

"Singing is breath," the third woman puts in. "And moving is life. So no wonder we start back from dancing!"

All three begin to talk, to laugh, as the two old hands welcome the new and begin to help her plan for living.

If you can't find the right family support group nearby, you might consider going to whatever family groups do exist in your area. Or ask the local chapter of your illness's national organization to try to set up a group. All you need guard against here is the old danger of getting too consumed by the illness. If that happens, quit. Until then, such groups can be wonderful.

# Chapter 13
## Joining the Club

Were the kids getting enough attention? During Seth's sophomore year at high school, one of his D & D friends spent a year out of town and Seth's little group of Bookies fell apart. He seemed lonely again, and unhappy. One day as I was putting rice into the turkey soup, he came into the kitchen and sat on a stool across the counter, his long, narrow face struggling to remain emotionless.

"Dad asked me to close the cur . . . tains in his study and when I didn't do it instantly, he got up and . . . *stumbled* across the room to close them. He stumbled on purpose! I know he did. It's . . . so awful!"

"It's hard. He does it to me, too." Commandment One: The mother must protect her children. Commandment Two: The mother must not bond with the son against the father. How to follow both commandments at once?

"I hate it when he does that!" Seth looked as helpless in his anger as Ted had years ago at the computer repair counter.

"Me too." The comforting smell of turkey soup wasn't going to be enough.

"Is that all you can say?"

"Sid and Mim were just saying to me how hard it must be for you. Perhaps it's hardest for you, to be growing up, to be becoming a man, as Dad is . . . well, getting weaker. And that's true. You do a good job. It's hard, isn't it?"

He started to say yes but had to stop.

I laid my hand on his. And then I blew it: "We have to imagine what it's like for him."

He straightened up and got red in the face: "He doesn't imagine what it's like for us!"

Ah, the justice of men. I couldn't answer. The mercy of women, perhaps, kept me from saying anything. So I said too little.

"You're in a tough spot." I failed my son.

One Sunday during eighth grade Debbie came home from an overnight, excited. I followed her upstairs and sat on her bed under the posters and beside our dog — the dog that rejoiced nightly at my arrival and never asked me the whereabouts of its blue jeans.

"It was *so* wonderful." She tossed dirty clothes out of her backpack. Her new haircut hung short over one ear and long over the other. At thirteen she prayed to reach fourteen and a half, the age at which we'd decreed she could pierce her ears.

"How come?" I patted our furry, good-smelling dog. There was something special about the look of enthusiasm on Debbie's too often saddened face; something in her had been really thrilled.

"There was a new girl and she talked about her father and how he had killed himself and I talked about Daddy."

"Oh, that's good." I touched the long side of her hair as she, too, sat down by the dog. "That's good."

What a thing for a thirteen-year-old to have to feel thrilled about! But at last, she'd found a dimension of change in a friend's life as staggering as the change in her own — indeed, more so. And she was talking. Nellie had noticed that Debbie's head often hung down. This new friendship might help her.

"That," said Debbie as we walked later in the meadow with the dog, "is what I'd paint if I were Nellie." She pointed to some wheat — simple, plain, and beautiful in form standing by a fence post.

"Or that." She pointed to the reflection of a cloud in a small puddle in the dirt road.

The dog ran at the far side of the meadow, after birds. She

seemed to fly, all four legs off the ground. She never came near to catching the birds; she never gave up trying.

"Next time, let's bring the camera down." I responded to this pleasure of Debbie's.

One Saturday, when Debbie was sick, I invited Seth to lunch at the Chinese restaurant. He'd always liked the one with the red-flocked wallpaper on Broadway in New York. It was our first grown-up lunch in that I felt for the first time the strain of intergenerational conversation. This is when I should be giving the pointers on life that my father used to give me.

"How's debating?" I picked up my chopsticks.

"Fine." He picked up his.

I had a lot to learn. Was it too late?

Firstborns tend to be academic and homebound like Seth. Secondborns tend to be social butterflies like Debbie. Theorists believe roles like that rigidify if there's stress in the family. But much of what the kids did seemed like ordinary teenage stuff. Ted thought I worried too much about them. He wasn't disposed to discuss them. Was that just a male reaction? Or a sick person's lack of energy? Or denial of trouble? Everything was so hard to sort out! How could I get the whole family doing things together again? First, I needed more for myself. I needed to exist again as myself alone. Dr. Feldman had set me on the way, but now I wanted the two-way street of friendship that therapy outlaws and parenting distorts and sickness makes hierarchical. I already had one nearby friend, Nellie.

"Smoking or nonsmoking?"

"Non!"

A waitress led Nellie and Nick and me to a table in the winter's sun. None of us had much money so we ordered cheaply and to share. It was the first time I'd eaten an ordinary business sort of lunch out in Highfield.

"So how's it going?"

We had our different answers. Both award-winning artists, Nellie and Nick were always short of cash. It was comforting to me to hear the trials of other free-lancers. Nellie was attempting to switch galleries in New York and Nick was expecting a visit from his former wife.

"Ted's on speed," I found myself saying for the first time.

"To get his muscles going in the morning. It makes him a little aggressive."

"My ex-wife did diet pills." Nick's blue eyes darkened. "She got very irritable."

"Volatile?"

"Very. Any little thing would set her off."

"Ted too, though he tries to be jolly. He always has some joke saved for when I get home. He swallows his words now. 'What?' I say. 'You're deaf,' he tells me abruptly. He's like a housewife who never gets out. I want to shout, 'For Pete's sake, couldn't you just wash the lettuce?' Actually, my husband cannot wash a head of lettuce. It requires a delicacy of finger control he does not possess. How can I get mad at that? I shouldn't say this. . . ."

"Talk." Nellie sat across the table next to Nick. Behind them waitresses moved among customers.

"Don't worry," Nick said. "We love Ted."

"Last night we had a fight. I'm lying there awake, mad. But that's bad. It could keep Ted awake. His lying awake could do damage to him. I can't have a problem of my own, the price is too high."

"It was like that with my wife," Nick said. "She wasn't a coper. I was her whole world. Somehow I had to keep her afloat all the time. I could never have the problem. She had them all. I couldn't take it."

"My husband considered himself a genius." Nellie finished her soup. "He didn't have time for anybody but himself."

So I wasn't the only one who didn't exist. Nellie and Nick had both divorced, though; I needed another way.

Outside the restaurant we hugged as we parted. Nick felt shorter but so much more stable than Ted, Nellie her warm self. When I climbed the stairs to my office, I felt accompanied, solidly there. My own emotions had been received, bounced back. Why couldn't Highfield be more like New York? In New York men and women ate lunch every day. The workplace allowed for male-female friendships laced with a mild flirtation. It was fun. I'd do it. Two of my magazine pieces had sold, and I began to eat lunch with Nick to talk about managing the free-lance life. And with Nellie to talk about art and the dedicated labor it demands. Then I began to collect more friends for lunches. The entertaining I did at home was mostly for Ted and the children; the lunches became mine. I wanted Ted to have friends other than me, too — friends to get news of the world from, a close friend to complain to, to shore him up. He'd always had friends in New York.

"Why don't you invite a friend for lunch or tea?"

"I need to save my energy for work." Ted and I sat wrapped like old people in afghans in his cold study, watching TV.

One day a young and beautiful admirer of Ted's Athens book came to interview him. I stopped work early and went cross-country skiing with Nick.

Nick pulled into a parking lot. Not me. Nick lifted out the skis. Not me. He waxed his and led off. He was a powerful skier. I had trouble keeping up. That in itself was wonderful. Under the stripped, dark trees I followed. It felt so good not to be in charge. We came to a pause at the top of a small hill.

"After a snow like this," he said, "I always think the world looks as it must have on creation day."

This was living as I remembered it. We even ate a chocolate bar. The sun even hung red over the snow.

At home, Ted's admirer was just leaving and Nellie was ringing the doorbell with a steaming pot of onion soup in her arms. Ted's visitor had told him his book was sensual.

"I tried not to stumble in her direction." He looked happy, refreshed.

It was Debbie's night to cook, and she was learning to broil chicken instead of warming up a pizza. All we had were two chicken breasts, but we cut them small and Nellie and Nick joined the four of us for supper at the round table in the room with the rosy velvet curtains: miracle of the loaves and fishes, things were multiplying.

"I feel surrounded by friends." Ted pulled the brown bedspread up to his nose. Other people's lives enclosed us like a shellfish's exoskeleton. We were protected. We began to feel slightly more normal, even though our own living tissue within had shrunken. No matter, we were together. Although I was learning to defuse myself from Ted in some ways, I would never take a lover. I wouldn't break open the basic tie of marriage. Socializing is enough; the dinner party was not got up by the Paleolithics for food alone. Friendship was the nourishment we needed, the children needed.

One day on the street, a woman from the writers' group stopped to talk about Ted.

"How can I help? I never know what to say to Ted about it."

"Take him for a ride some afternoon, to that old mill off the highway, maybe?"

We parted and I started up my office stairs. There was plenty that friends could do. They wanted to help Ted but were scared. Maybe they'd put a foot in their mouths if they mentioned his illness. Or maybe they wondered whether he'd fall over if they touched him. The woman hadn't asked how she could help me, but people often did and I never could think of anything specific. I rolled paper into my typewriter and tapped out some pages telling how friends actually can help all the members of a family where there is chronic illness. My agent thought it might sell and that I should draft the article.

I interviewed Ted first, as we were driving to his neurologist's.

"Tell them not to grab doors to open for people with canes," he said. "Half the time I'm leaning on the door. I lose my balance."

I pulled into the handicapped parking space and we walked slowly together, negotiating the doctor's carpet. We sat opposite a blond man whose wife sat in a wheelchair. He looked dead of desire.

As Ted settled himself in his chair, I got out my notebook.

"Everybody asks me how I'm feeling." Ted lifted his right leg up into place. "What can I say? I'm lousy? I wish they'd forget about sickness and just ask me if I saw the Celtics game. I'm bored with being sick. I want to be myself, my essential self."

"What about calling friends? Why don't you call friends more?"

"I need my energy for work." His curly hair was receding fast, but his light eyes remained as kindly as ever. "I guess it's more than that, though." He sat forward and slowly maneuvered his way out of his puffy jacket.

"I just don't have any . . . initiative. If they want to be friends, I'm glad. But sometimes I don't call back. So tell them not to be hurt if a sick friend doesn't call back. Keep trying."

The nurse was opening the inner door.

"And it'd be good if Nick would take me to the post office.

I'd like to buy my own stamps without asking you. Or Nellie could take me to the antique store. You hate to go. Oh, I know, the worst thing . . . tell them not to tell their sick friends that their tiredness is just middle age."

"Ted!" The nurse lost a chance to dignify her patient with a mister. After he started to walk toward her, she called the woman in the wheelchair.

The blond man wheeled his wife in and returned to his seat. He picked up a magazine. He flipped a page. His life-suspended expression didn't change. Was there such a thing as a well spouse expression? Such a thing as a well spouse syndrome?

I interviewed Seth when he stopped by my office to tell me he'd set aside some new jeans and a sweater. Could I pick them up on my credit card? Since the article was slanted toward how friends could help, I asked him what our friends could do for him, considering his dad was sick.

His face broke into a smile. "Buy me a stereo!"

I interviewed Debbie as we drove to her flute lesson. She challenged family tradition by playing a musical instrument.

I gave her the same question and got the same answer.

With her hair over one eye, she smiled: "Buy me a stereo!"

"They're okay," I assured Ted under the brown bedspread. "All they want is stereos."

We laughed and held hands. Since Ted could scarcely feel my hand with his right, he switched to his left.

*Woman's Day* took my piece. Month after month, they didn't schedule it. "It's a downer," my editor there explained. A downer? How could it be, it was so specific about how to help. I opened a copy of the magazine to a piece by a woman out west who'd adopted something like fourteen mentally and/or physically handicapped children. She was having a dandy time.

That summer when Seth was cleaning clams in his first job and Debbie had gone to New York alone on a bus, I picked up my old college friend Angela and her husband, Ben, from the Boston bus. She'd called to say they'd be in the area for a conference. Ben plunged down the steps of the bus, controlling his Parkinson legs from somewhere not quite right in his brain. He didn't fall. Angela came next carrying three heavy bags, her blond hair tucked up in a becoming knot. They were just back from Spain where Ben — once a world-class biologist — had been lecturing.

"He looks pretty good," I told Angela a few minutes later in my sunny kitchen, as I sliced cheese on a board.

"He's awful." She tucked a pin in her hair. "Spain was terrible. I was always carrying two suitcases in one hand and trying to hail a taxi with the other while wondering if he'd fallen over the curb. Ted doesn't look so great either. How is he?"

"He's been exacerbating. Summer."

Angela put her arms around me by the sink. "If we didn't love them," she said, "we would hate them."

At the dining room table, Ben sat big and immobile in his chair. Ted was talking. They weren't really talking to each other. It looked like parallel play. Angela and I laughed at everybody's jokes, brought in courses, and cleaned up. Then we went for a walk in the meadow.

What had happened to all those men Angela and I had sewn the pinnies for? Stalks of corn grew, taller than Angela or me, and the summer insects hummed in ways significant to themselves. Dust rose around us as we walked. I told Angela about my article and found myself asking, "What's it like for you, living with the illness?"

"There's no room for me! No room at all." Angela walked steadily beside me in the heat. "No physical space, no psychic space, nothing."

"Me too!" I felt suddenly lightfooted. "Exactly. No room."

"The other day I was saying to a friend that if I were Ben I'd have jumped out the window by now." Angela kicked at a pebble in the dirt road without breaking stride. "She said something surprising. She said if she were *me*, she'd have jumped out by now."

Aah. We walked, silently through the dust, unsure just how much we wanted to reveal.

"He won't do anything," Angela went on carefully, kicking a pebble. "Nothing, not one thing. He reads and writes, but he won't do the bills, even if he says he's going to. He walks along Boston Common and shops for ice cream for himself, but he won't pick up his shoes from the repairman."

"Yes." I looked around at the sky, the cornfield, the rising dust. "Ted promised to call a man to get an estimate on the porch roof fourteen months ago." I kicked at a pebble, too.

So we were together. Kicking at stones, we walked on in the buzz of summer.

"Nothing! He won't do a Goddamned thing. I have to do everything. And I mean everything, every single thing!" In Angela's loudening voice that faded safely in the dusty space, I could hear my own hidden intonations.

A therapist might say, "Hey, wait a minute." But Angela and I knew what we knew and we each needed to hear our feelings validated, guilt-free. It felt so good to hear somebody corroborating my own reality. When she spoke, I could hear how justified her feelings were. Not that her feelings were the whole picture. But they were a part, a valid part. I knew she loved Ben. She knew I loved Ted. And there on the road kicking stones, we each discovered how annoyed and disappointed and lonely and squelched and tired we both were. Clearly there was a well spouse syndrome.

On the far side of the cornfields, we walked under the trees to the river and sat in the dank coolness.

"So what's your average day like?"

"I'm at work, say." Angela quieted, sounding matter-of-fact. "It's midafternoon, I know Ben's helper will be leaving any minute. Maybe he's left. I sit at my desk. I start trying not to phone home. Because if I do phone home and he doesn't answer, I panic. So for a couple of hours, I don't call. Then it's five and I sit on the T wondering what I'll find when I get to Cambridge. He could be dead. He could have fallen and broken a bone. He could be stuck on the couch, sitting with his mouth open, unable to move. Or he could just be watching television. Maybe mumbling a little about things that aren't there."

"Hallucinations?" I picked a small stone from the bank and pitched it into the river. Light came dappled over the rocks, the ferny bank.

"Sort of. Fears. A little of this, a little of that. I stop at the store and pick up some groceries and then it's under the arbor and into the building. I unlock the door and look into the living room. Ah, there he is. It's okay. Not dead. Just stuck, can't get up off the couch alone. I put the groceries down and go to him. Heave a little, ho a little, and he's up. When that's over, I carry the groceries into the kitchen. Newspaper all every which way over the kitchen table or the floor. Apple cores on the floor. An empty carton of ice cream on the table. He is a slob. A slob! I mean, it's repulsive. Just to look at a place where he's been! So

I pick up the apple cores and the dripping carton and I put away the groceries. Then, if he's bad, we move into the bedroom."

Angela tried to skid a flat stone along the water.

"It's like a jail in that bedroom. We live in that bedroom. It, too, is a mess. Bits of food on the floor. I pick up. I get myself a drink to kill the pain, to relax, to stop being mad. I drink, we watch the news. Then I broil the chicken, make a salad. I cook less and less. Really, in the last few years I don't do much but broil chicken or scramble some eggs and a salad. I have to say, he's always happy to eat whatever I make. In some ways, he's a saint. It's awful. He never complains. I can't stand it. I do all his complaining for him. I hate it. We eat in front of the TV because he seldom talks anymore. All those wonderful things he knows and he never talks anymore! Except when people come or when we go out."

Strange, startling, the similarities. I leaned back to put my face up into the splotchy light.

"By then it's nine or so and I'm tired. I clean up. If he's not talking, I usually just fall asleep while he's watching television. I go to bed before ten, exhausted. Then the night begins. He wakes me four or five times a night because he gets stuck. A leg falls out of the bed; he can't move his arm. Or he gets scared and shouts, "Get out of the bed! I'm going to explode!" My alarm rings at six and I get up to swim at the Y. I have to keep fit. How else will I be strong enough to move him? Besides, swimming's fun. It's for me. Me! I'm okay at my desk till afternoon. Then at just about the time his helper leaves, I start to get anxious again. At five on the dot I leave. While I'm heading out of the building, somebody usually passes me near the elevators and says solicitously . . ." — here Angela lowered her voice and leaned toward me — " 'How's *Ben?*' "

We laughed, holding our knees, rocking backward.

How freeing these terrible words were for me. Just to have them spoken. To hear them without having to focus my sympathies on Ben. Just to let the other side, Angela's and mine, into the light. To let it be, without apology, without guilt. There was a well spouse syndrome and this was it.

"We should talk more!"

Refreshed, we stood up from the river and began the walk home. We resolved to try to get out one night a week each, to meet halfway on the highway between us for dinner, to keep each other posted. Back in the house, we went into the separate bedrooms where our husbands were resting. Ted was lying in the air conditioning, losing his left hand.

"What a wonderful life we have," Ted said. "What wonderful friends. We have a wonderful life, despite everything. It's wonderful. Turn the cooler to low."

He didn't say please.

After Angela and Ben left, I ran into a woman downtown whom Ted and I had met at an MS Society meeting. Maybe I could talk well-spouse-ese to her. "Sometimes I get a little discouraged," I began. "Do you, ever?"

"No." She stood impassive.

Guilt-struck, I realized this wouldn't be easy.

In my office, I called the MS Society. They said they'd never been able to raise a spouse support group in our area. I called the paper and ran an ad for an MS spouse support group. It came out right under Al-Anon's ad. Weeks later, my office phone rang. A distraught woman said she'd been saving my ad for the moment when she couldn't hang on any longer. Could she join the group? I had to confess that it was just her and me and maybe one other woman. So Maggie's Folly met at my office: I borrowed chairs and lamps; how strange my white office looked at night.

Helen's husband had just been forced to retire. He sat all day watching C-span. Twenty years ago he'd been outgoing; today he is depressed. Sometimes she would go into the garage and turn on the lawn mower and mow the backyard so she could cry. She didn't want him to know she was frightened. It would scare him.

Maureen's husband still worked. He'd just gone into Canadian crutches and was thrilled to be off her arm. What she missed most was going out at night, to the movies, to dinner, to concerts.

Here it was, the well spouse experience. But that's as far as we could get. We couldn't talk about ourselves. We'd gotten into the habit of looking to our sick for drama. If any of us accidentally brushed against our own drama or our own anger, we apologized instantly and profusely. We were good girls trying to remain good.

There was factual exchange: all three men had experienced exaggerated responses to weather for decades; all three had found trouble balancing the checkbook but hung on so as not to feel emasculated — while checks bounced and all three wives sweated it out. One husband seemed to be having trouble hearing and he, too, told his wife she must be deaf.

"I re-spond by spea-king ve-ry clear-ly," she demonstrated. "And by turn-ing to face him in ev-er-y dir-ec-tion. He never turns to face me."

Oh, yes. This was it, even our speech was altered to meet their needs. But the group came to an end after a few sessions because we couldn't be bad, couldn't be mad. Did we need a leader to give us permission? Perhaps Angela was a fluke? Perhaps *Woman's Day* would never run my piece? And if they did, would I get hate mail?

The piece ran and heartfelt letters arrived, surprisingly not from the friends of the chronically ill but from their wives:

"Dear Maggie," wrote a woman from Florida. "I feel that I know you well enough to call you by your first name. What a relief to read about another family who is going through the same experiences. . . ."

A wife from California: "You have no idea how much the writing of your life . . . meant to us. It was comforting to know that we are not unique."

From Michigan: "I cried and cried, so did my husband. I hadn't cried yet — not for the diagnosis — not for my husband — not for the kids — not even for myself — but your article made me realize all the things, experiences, friends, that we no longer can have. By admitting that things are different and accepting this illness — I have come around the corner to adjust myself and the children. Until now, I've been going at such a fast pace to make everything as normal . . . ."

From Kansas: "I am tired of catheters, suppositories, lifting, pushing, fetching, sarcasm, demands, cutting words, mood swings . . . I thank you for your article because you were able to show the family side of chronic illness."

From New York: "I think this is the first 'fan letter' I've ever written to an author! Thank you for such straightforward advice. Perhaps you're also working on a book on the subject?"

A book. I'd long wanted Ted and me to write a double book with alternating chapters on the sick experience and the well experience. He'd refused. I tried him one last time.

"No," he said, in the kitchen where I was baking apples. "I

don't want to write about sickness. You write it alone. I'll write the sequel. I'll call it *Ted Gets Well*."

Okay, I'd write just for us well spouses, then. We needed each other. Therapy helped (sometimes) and friends helped, but there was nothing quite like my talk with Angela, nothing like having our combined servant and master role spoken aloud, verified. With help from others who needn't apologize or explain, from men and women who knew the same shorthand, we all might gather energy for life.

The kids said okay.

But should I? Did I really want to spend a couple of years thinking about degenerative illnesses?

Water ran on the slickery streets. The phone rang in my office. It was Francie, making her first continental call. Did I remember her from the stress conference in Chicago? Of course I remembered her! She told how her husband had felt sick at the airport as they saw their child off to college. How the dialysis shunt had developed a low-grade infection. How he'd required surgery and that he was out of his mind with depression. How she'd been driving back and forth from Pasadena to the university hospital across Los Angeles traffic while worrying if he were passing out beside her, or bleeding internally.

"I've lost my tolerance for masochism," she concluded. "You've been doing it for six years. How can you stand it?"

"I can't," I told her. "None of us can."

So I decided to write this book.

# Chapter 14
# Acts of Rescue (And What About That Affair?)

Sooner or later we stand back from the illness, back from the man or woman we've married, back from the children, and wonder as everyone does after too many dark days, "Who am I?" Too often the well spouse's answer comes in a whisper: "I'm sad and angry and too wrung out to know."

How do you build a new, in some ways more single, life out of the dust of the chronic emotions? Psychiatrist Dr. Clara Livsey, formerly of the Sinai Hospital in Baltimore, speaks on the telephone from Berkeley.

"I emphasize finding sources of pleasure. I've had people reject that idea, say 'Are you telling me to have fun at this terrible moment?' But that moment is life." Dr. Livsey goes on to explain that each person in a couple is different, although couples are, to some degree, emotionally fused. "The more you can become unfused and the more outlets and pleasure you can find, the more you have energy and love and emotions to give to the person who is disabled." It shouldn't come as a surprise that Dr. Livsey has lived with a chronic condition: she moved to Berkeley to be near her quadriplegic son, who wished to make use of the city's Center for Independent Living.

How to start? Dr. Livsey suggests by "putting a certain distance between yourself and the sick one. Explain to the sick person that you'll function better if you take care of yourself. You must build a life of your own."

Where do well spouses themselves report finding separate pleasures? What really works?

### EXERCISE

This tops the well spouse list for a surefire self-helping act. It makes sense: muscular exertion turns off the body's "get-ready-to-run-or-fight" response to stress. In upstate New York, Laurie jogs:

> There will be days when only that three-mile run or aerobics class or an hour session on the Nautilus machine can keep you from the depths of total depression. If you have been exercising and playing sports regularly, don't give them up. Your spouse (if he's as wonderful a person as mine is) will understand that having time to yourself for recreation and exercise is as vital as his or her medications or therapy.

### RELAXATION TECHNIQUES

Using an opposite approach, Yoga and meditation techniques demonstrate how to still the body and still the mind, how to turn off that great anxious planner in your head. A woman from Vermont:

> I go to Yoga one night a week. I go in tense and caught up in my lists: are we packed for the next chemo, when is the man coming to fix the floor, how will I read fifty class papers over the weekend? We stretch and bend and listen to our instructor's soothing voice telling us to let go of self-judgment and let go of responsibility. Well, it falls right away. She leads us into a deep relaxation, and lying there on the floor in the dark I usually feel tears in my eyes. It's good. I lie there and the tears roll out of the corners of my eyes and then she brings tea and turns on the light and I feel terrific, relaxed! I sleep better than any other night. My lists don't start up again until the morning.

### SLOW IS BEAUTIFUL

Here are ten instructions Dr. Meyer Friedman (see Appendix B), director of the Recurrent Coronary Prevention Project at the Mount Zion Hospital in downtown San Francisco, gives his coronary patients. In the early 1980s, he and his colleague Dr.

Carl Thoreson, a professor of education at Stanford University, used an extended version of this list (along with a program of diet and exercise) with 592 men who'd had heart attacks. Only 7 percent of the men suffered another attack. It doesn't matter here if this program actually prevents heart attacks. What matters is how these ten habits can help a person who lives under inavoidable stress to relax. I've dubbed them Slow Is Beautiful. Try:

> *To walk more slowly.*
> *To talk more slowly.*
> *To eat more slowly.*
> *To play games to lose, not win.*
> *To write down whatever makes you angry.*
> *To smile at others' foibles.*
> *To laugh at yourself.*
> *To do one thing at a time.*
> *To admit you're wrong.*
> *To stop interrupting.*

Personally, I find that these help. Here's what happened when I tried them. Walking slower, I found that my posture improved. Walking became "being" instead of "getting somewhere." Surprisingly, my vision changed, too. It was as if my gaze came back into my body and no longer spun out, overextended. I stopped planning what to buy everybody for Christmas. I drew back into myself. Time broke into smaller bits and each bit lasted longer.

Talking slower, I became more truthful and used blunter words. There was less to say. I stopped repeating myself.

That's just the beginning. Try the rest yourself.


CUTTING THE BOOZE

Alcohol is one of the most common palliatives that we well spouses, along with the rest of the race, take for sorrow, boredom, stress, and fear. Like us, widows are noted for it.

There's a connection (expressed in chemicals) between depression and alcoholism. What makes you sensitive to sadness may also make you crave alcohol. The more you drink, the emotionally emptier you may feel — since alcohol takes the edge off all emotions, not just sorrow.

According to the *University of California, Berkeley, Wellness Letter* (see Appendix B), published monthly in association with the School of Public Health, a 160-pound man can drink no more than 5 ounces of wine, 12 ounces of beer, or 1½ ounces of hard liquor an hour without having it build up toward drunkenness. Once the alcohol from a drink is absorbed into the bloodstream, it takes the body about an hour to dispose of it. Every drink, as previously defined, puts about two-thirds of an ounce of pure alcohol into the bloodstream. If a 120-pound woman drinks three 5-ounce glasses of wine in two hours at a party, it will build her blood alcohol level to .09. Most states start drunk driving levels at .10.

Small doses of alcohol or none mean that your evenings stretch out longer and that you force yourself to learn to fill them in more varied ways.

### GET YOUR SLEEP

The double bed stands for adulthood, marriage, and the nightly comfort of being a pair. Few of us want to leave it. But the sick may wake often and get up frequently and sleep restlessly. It's very hard to break the double bed tie. The sick feel abandoned. The well feel ambivalent and guilty. The greatest blessing a sick spouse could give here would be to say, "Let's get twin beds. You need your sleep." But if your spouse can't do this, sit down and resolve your own ambivalence. When you're ambivalent, it's hard to stick to your decisions. You're a pushover for anyone with a stronger opinion. Make up your mind. Stick to it.

You can always push the single beds together.

Spouses nursing the very sick may need single rooms.

If you're still not sleeping, cut caffeine and alcohol. If that doesn't work, get help. "Don't live with chronic insomnia," says psychiatrist and sleep specialist Dr. Quentin Regestein (see Appendix B).

### CHECK OUT WORRIES ABOUT YOUR HEALTH

You're vulnerable to the stress-related illnesses. Check into any variances: pain, changes in eating or drinking or sleeping, changes in urine or bowels, headaches, "funny" sensations, weight loss or gain, vision or hearing problems, dizziness.

Sure, we're all hypochondriacs. Don't feel embarrassed. We've seen illness at first hand. We're scared. It's a further drain to be worrying about a possible illness of our own. Make a doctor's appointment. While you wait, check out what's bothering you by calling the Tel Medex at your hospital or by asking the research librarian to direct you to a useful medical encyclopedia. Of course, you can drive yourself wild researching symptoms. But a nagging worry drives you wild, too. Go to the doctor whenever you want reassurance. Tell him you live under unusual stress and need to stop worrying. The husband of a woman who's had breast cancer says:

> I go every year. "So what is it this year?" my doctor says. We've been through colon cancer, arthritis, lung cancer, and arteriosclerosis. Actually, I'm fine. I usually feel pretty good for a few months after I see the doctor. Then I start to worry and make an appointment for several months ahead. That gives whatever it is time to go away and yet I feel I'm doing the right thing by myself to look into it.

### Is It Menopause?

Insomnia, fatigue, headache, and irritability are all listed under menopause's symptoms. Of course, these may be run-of-the-mill symptoms of the overtaxed well wife. They may also be the symptoms of the very illnesses well spouses are prone to. Which is which?

A well wife's normal aging looks like Easy Street to her superaging husband: sickness, in a sense, is speeded-up aging. Once again, needs may not be met at home. If you've got a sense of humor, it may be fun to find a friend whose teeth are also growing brittle and whose hair is also drying out. She'll help you sort out which of your symptoms come from menopause and which don't. For more expert opinion, of course, talk with your gynecologist.

### Travel Around the Emotional Wheel

Psychologists do not even agree yet on the basic emotions or how we come by them. Some even think that an exterior show of emotions — such as that produced by placing the facial muscles into arrangements resembling how we look when we feel certain ways — can actually make us feel those ways. Jump up and down for joy and smile. Do you feel better?

One well spouse sent me this wheel of simple emotions and said she tries to get all the way around it every day.

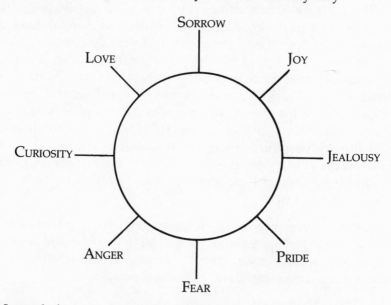

I watch for any sign of the happier emotions. Curiosity is the easiest. Everytime I feel curious, I stop what I'm doing and try to follow the feeling and enjoy it. Pride is possible, too. I'm proud of myself, of being able to live this life. I'm proud of my kids, of my husband, too. I'm proud of the United States of America, the great dream of the nation, Martin Luther King's dream. Love comes, off and on. I feel it around me when I'm walking down the street on a good day — the young mothers with their babies in the strollers, the fathers with their babies on their backs. I'm touched by old people looking straight ahead. By boys walking in groups. I love them all! The whole human race. It's catchy. Joy, that's the toughest, though it comes right up out of the others. I don't get there too often. The more I walk among trees the closer I get. Days that I get all the way around the wheel, I know I'm alive.

### SET TRAPS FOR THOSE LIGHTER EMOTIONS

That woman's wheel increases awareness. You can set traps for the lighter emotions by using her wheel or by increasing exposure to the things you like. In 1985, Dr. Avram Goldstein, a phar-mapsychologist at Stanford University — interested in the pos-sibility that sudden, strong emotions correlate with abrupt drops or rises in body chemicals — asked 250 people what gave them a thrill. The top seven thrillers: music; a good movie; beauty in nature or art; physical contact with another person; a climactic moment in an opera; and (tied) sex and nostalgic moments.

What thrills you? Poetry? Kids? Parades? How can you pro-vide yourself with more exposure to these pleasurable things?

Start small. Francie passed what she called the perfect bumper sticker for the well spouse on the highway outside L.A. It said, "Have a nice moment." Plan some small daily reward that gives you something to look forward to. Keep the emphasis on small. Yearning for the unrealistic (three weeks in the Caribbean with the perfect lover) will only hurt more.

Laurie sums it up:

> No matter how bad your situation gets, try hard to find something to be happy about. It could be as simple as the bright flight of a cardinal to your snow-covered backyard bird feeder. Hang on to something good, something positive.

## IMAGINE HAPPY OUTCOMES

Either in response to our sick spouses' denial or simply in response to our situations, we tend to start expecting the next blow. Instead, try to imagine things turning out well, small things — we're not moving mountains here. Here's a man whose wife suffered a stroke:

> When I'm driving along and start to get tense or worried, I tell myself to "relax behind the eyes. It's going to be okay." I just say those words and something does change around my eyes and I begin to picture the best outcome of whatever task I'm engaged in. The music at the supermarket won't be on too loud, I'll be able to find the capers.

## RELIGION

The established religions help millions of people. There's the social element and then there is the deep rest in something larger, the profound trust that everything does, indeed, turn out the way a (hopefully) benign force wishes it. It works for Jill:

I just pray, a lot, for the answers that I don't have. My faith in God (and my daughter) keep me moving forward.

If the established religions aren't for you, take a broader look. However you put it together, your view of the world is, in a sense, your religion. Resolving your personal worldview matters enormously. As one woman put it: "I get a nice bunch of people at the Unitarian Church and I get my spiritual contact when I garden."


TEMPORARY FLIGHT

First, there's the simple need to get away from the sickness. Then there's the need to learn to be alone, to find out who you are beyond being a member of a pair. You're not single, but you're not quite married the way you were, either. Who are you?

Take nights out. Weekends off. Weeks away. This is easier for the spouse who already believes that a marriage consists of two separate individuals. Men or women in extremely cohesive marriages who think of themselves as incomplete without their spouses will have to start very small. They will require a lot of encouragement.

An independent woman, Francie finds it easier — although it took her a year to do the following:

I go out to a café a couple of blocks away maybe twice a month, alone. I sit at a table and drink club soda and listen to the singer. Once in a while I sit at the bar and drink a glass of wine. Sometimes I talk back to the men who open conversations with me. That's all I do. It's a great relief, just to be out, away alone, being myself alone away from home. The person I am with Eric is not my entire self. Nobody is her entire self or his entire self with a spouse. And the day will come when Eric won't be here. I need to know that I can survive that. Already, I've split in two: one part of me tries to save him and be with him, the other part tries to remember who I am and to save me.

Kathy reports simple breaks for the comfort of solitude:

I live five minutes from sand and salt water. Though I've never gone alone to the movies, I go to the beach alone — just sit and sift! It's a regenerating experience. I take walks, lots of walks.

Leaving or staying in a marriage is based on the whole personality, the whole relationship, and the whole context of the life together, not on the specific quality of sexual life. Yet well spouses who deal with a reduced sexual life miss sex a great deal. If they confess to it, friends and therapists forever ask, "Why don't you have an affair?"

Some give religious answers. "Me? I'm Catholic!" "Me? I'm born again!" Others say, "If I break this basic bond, this basic privacy, where will I draw the line?" When death is near, allegiance runs too high to raise the question. If spouses do look for a nice easy sexual connection just to make them feel alive again, they seem to find it's not so easy. Here are their reasons:

*Depletion.* They're too tired. Physically and emotionally exhausted. They really haven't anything to offer anyone. All they can do is take, and who's giving?

*Age.* Women say it's hard enough for single women in their forties and fifties to find sexual companions. Men mention a reduced desire and sometimes a fear of impotence.

*Fear of rejection.* The age-old male/female fear.

*Lack of time.* Time to think Who? Time to court. Time to get away.

*Lack of money.* Many well spouses haven't got the dough for a decent haircut, never mind wine or roses or money for a babysitter.

*Isolation from the opposite sex.* Women engaged in home nursing seldom get out at all. Men filling in at home curtail other social functions.

*Sexual programming.* Middle-aged women were brought up when the boys telephoned the girls. A married woman with a sick husband has to be able to make it perfectly clear to a possible sexual companion that she is available: many can't. Men programmed to let women handle emotional connection may feel entirely closed off by the reduced intimacy at home. To open up to any woman might mean they'd abandon the sick spouse, and so they hold back.

*Maternal or paternal programming from the situation itself.* One woman told me that she felt attracted to a man at a wedding, and after they danced she patted him on the shoulder because she'd been taking care of her husband and children so long she'd forgotten how to do anything else.

*They may have put sexuality into deep freeze.* As discussed in chapter 8, once this happens it's really tough to get thawed out.

*They're unapproachable.* People think of well spouses as saints. And they fear to tread on sick mates' territory — out of the same guilt we all feel toward the sick.

Can't it be done?

Cammy managed to have an affair. She's now an attractive and self-possessed woman of thirty-eight. Here's what happened:

> He was someone who had always flirted with me at my office and I with him. He didn't intersect with either my work life or my family life. Not at all. So he was safe. I couldn't afford anything else. He was insistent. That was a prerequisite, I guess. I put him through a lot of courting, a lot of flirtation.
>
> And then one day, I just knew I would go along with it. I can't say I made up my mind ahead of time. We went to his apartment. I was still deciding, still prettily protesting, you could say. So then it began.
>
> He was married. I knew I wasn't his first extramarital affair. Yet he wasn't exactly a womanizer. It was wonderful, in a way. It got me through a couple of very bad years. But it wasn't an answer.
>
> I found out I really can't handle recreational sex. After years of living with my husband's sickness, I had enormous emotional needs. So an affair wasn't the answer for me — I couldn't afford to let things complexify emotionally. I just couldn't handle any more complications. I couldn't handle another part of my life, another area, in which I had no control. When you are powerless at home against the illness and then you let somebody else into your life, you are opening yourself to being at somebody's mercy in another sphere. It's too much. You can't go on performing those small performances romance requires.
>
> There certainly was a definite limitation to what I could offer this man and there was a limitation to what he could offer me, too. After a while, I decided I'd rather have nobody.

Is it easier for men? Here's a man's report:

> I haven't done it or contemplated it. I don't want to go outside my marriage. I guess now, looking back, whatever gets you through the night is okay. . . . But maybe you just can't do it all. You reach limits. In my case, it's an issue over time and energy.

In a crass sense, I'm a good commodity. It wouldn't be hard for me to have an affair in terms of finding somebody. But what kind of woman would want to get involved with me? I don't have enough energy for it.

Doesn't it ever work?

Here's one well husband's story told not by him but by the "other woman." She was unhappily married and got divorced in the course of the story. We have to imagine Bruce's version.

I bumped into Bruce on Park Avenue one summer evening. He'd done some work for my company once and was in town for the week, so we had dinner. We stayed in the restaurant till they closed the doors at 2:30 A.M. and took a cab to my apartment. We were shaking, both of us. We'd fallen in love. But nothing happened. The next day, we met for lunch and he made it clear that he was a devoted husband. His wife had had a stroke ten years earlier and had no sexual interest in him. But she was a dear woman and a fine mother. He worked, worked, and worked. The two kids were about to go to college.

For about four months, we had lunch or cocktails. He felt guilty about what he was doing to me and what he was doing to his wife. He would never divorce her. He couldn't stand it. We tried breaking up regularly. We would both cry and start over again. We were walking on a cloud. Finally, he came to my apartment.

Sex started poorly, we felt so guilty. But we bought books. We conquered that. Our love was very strong, unbelievably fulfilling. He always left my place and went back to his hotel room to check for messages from his wife. He even mussed up the bed. He called her every night and she was a big talker, too. None of his friends knew about me. All my friends knew about him.

Bruce had married while he and his wife were still in college. He'd never dated anyone else. He said he'd never known what it was like to be madly in love. Over and over, he said that if he died tomorrow, he had lived. The affair lasted seventeen years. He left all his worldly goods to his wife. She never found out. Even now I feel strangely guilty writing about this, but I know that she certainly had a much happier husband than she would have had otherwise.

THERE'S ALWAYS A DOG

This woman writes from New Hampshire:

One other thing. We bought a dog for the girls some five years ago. Hazel has listened to more complaints and fears, seen more tears — and has never been anything more than the most faithful, caring friend. If you don't have one, get a pet. Get a cat or a dog. Something you can hold . . . cry into . . . say terrible things to. It's wonderful therapy.

## A Good Job Is Best

If you don't already work outside the home, why not? Work satisfies, and being away from the sickness helps, as do the friendships of the workplace. Kathy reports:

> My work is my sanity. It takes me away from my pain and gives me a break. I have such support from my colleagues. At work I'm glad they don't ask daily how Sandy is — it's boring to talk about it. Yet a meal is brought when I need it, somebody's husband helps fix my car, another's does my taxes, another takes over at my desk if I have to run for a prescription.
>
> Which brings us to the very foundation of the new individual life — friends.

## And Friends

Of course, a friend made for a purpose isn't a friend. The point is that there are all kinds of love, and friendship is one kind — we need to be nurtured by love. Our sick spouses love us and we love them, but often the love is altered by demands of illness.

This is a good decade for friendship because there are so many single people. They have lots of energy and they need friends as much as we do. Make your friends into a kind of family.

You need friends who can respond to you emotionally with the full panoply that the sick find hard to sustain. Miriam says:

> For friends, I have Tess. She likes to give gifts — a floral potpourri, scented body lotion. But she also gives herself, her humor, her vitality. She understands depression, fear, and sadness. Last spring she stopped in unexpectedly. Our house was a way station at that time on her emotional highway. She looked wonderful in her bright red, puffed-sleeved jacket, but

she needed to talk about something troubling her. We circled our acre of garden and weeds, noticing crocuses and snow-drops, talking, crying, laughing. A wonderful moment of support and trust. I do love Tess: she nurtures me.

You need friends to corroborate your experience and keep you in touch with your own sanity — it goes too easily out of kilter if the sick deny reality.

You need friends to discuss problems with, the problems that for one reason or another cause division at home. Money, perhaps, or a situation with a child that demands energy for research and discussion. Divert only those things that you and your spouse cannot learn to deal with — otherwise, you take too much out of the twosome.

You need friends simply to do healthly things with, such as mountain climbing or canoeing or dancing or staying up late or walking in the woods or swimming. Don't they sound good?

You need friends to give you practical help, such as raking leaves and putting in the storm windows and carting off the old basketball hoop and picking up a kid stranded at a hockey game and delivering the balloons to the birthday party. Says Tom in Houston:

> There is a friend of Lisa's who is incredible, an upbeat but realistic person. Some people are upbeat to the extent of being unreal. They turn everything into a heroic struggle. This person is very matter-of-fact and does a lot of little pragmatic things. That's what you need.

And you need friends to keep the whole family floating in a social network.

Watch out at the start: you may be so desperate that you demand too much from friends.


### Make Friends Out of Family

Perhaps you are close with your family and your spouse's. This is rare in our mobile century. Some people go through life talking ritually with in-laws but not quite as themselves. Look over your entire extended family — are there people with whom you could become real friends?

For the long haul, imagine living two lives — one among friends and one at home. This is apples and oranges again. You will feel torn apart sometimes, but for many of us it's preferable to feeling permanently trapped and isolated.

The sick spouse finally accepts that he's sick and begins to adjust. He or she makes the best of things. The well spouse joins in that process and is part of it. But the well spouse also lives in the well world and must accept that. The well spouse always remains partly divided. We hold ourselves together by taking ourselves apart, by fragmenting. Be whole and well in the world. You are not sick. You are not sick. You are not sick.

# Chapter 15
## How Are the Kids?

Ted's left leg got tired compensating for his right and he was having more and more trouble walking. His neurologist mentioned Cytoxan, a chemotherapy that early studies warned might produce leukemia ten years later in perhaps a quarter of its recipients. I begged Ted not to try it. His father had just been diagnosed with leukemia, the good kind, slow. Wouldn't this put Ted into the worst brackets?

"Wait a minute," Ted said when Seth tried to turn the TV channel. "They're showing something about a new treatment for leukemia, and I want to see it in case I take Cytoxan."

"What?"

"Cytoxan. It's a drug I might take for MS. Sometimes it causes leukemia."

"I'm against that!" Almost sixteen, Seth sat tall on the couch and wrapped himself, including his face, in one of the afghans even though it was April. "Don't take that!"

"I want to make up my own mind." Ted leaned forward to catch the televised words.

"What's this?" Debbie, almost fourteen, came out of her bedroom.

"A report on leukemia." Ted leaned still farther forward.

"Oh." She sat on the arm of the couch and swung her leg back and forth.

The dog shuffled into the room and lay down. On the screen, doctors told an older man in California that he could sustain no more chemotherapy. Between camera shots, two years passed while they gave him monoclonic antibodies specific to his kind of leukemia. We saw him again, older, thinner, but clearly healthier. He was climbing up onto a boat, his boat. The treatment cost about fifty thousand dollars and wasn't covered by insurance.

"Don't do it," Seth said, his voice muffled by the afghan. "I don't want you to do that."

"Me neither," I joined in. "Don't do it."

"Do what?" Debbie stopped swinging her leg.

Ted cleared his throat. "Take a drug that might keep me walking longer. It could give me leukemia later, maybe ten years down the road."

"You?" Debbie cried, putting her arm around Ted's neck. "I thought you were talking about Grandpa!"

So we all sat around the couch, holding hands, not talking. We were so quiet, so connected, that the dog ran up and tried to get into the circle the way she does when we hug each other or sing "Happy Birthday."

Except for Tuesday afternoons when a friend drove him, Ted hadn't left the house without me in two years. I wanted him to get an Amigo. It's a battery-driven wheelchair that looks like a golf cart. He could go downtown alone. He could get a haircut without me. He could even make it into the accessed library. Besides, a nurse had warned me that some people with MS wake up one day unable to walk — it's best to have your systems in place.

"It's too soon." Ted sat on the porch at twilight.

"Just for outdoors?" I breathed in the sixth season of lilacs.

"Okay. I'll rent one and see." He looked wistfully through the screen.

The rented Amigo came on the Friday of Memorial Day weekend and sat unremarked in the farthest end of the living room. The children didn't want to acknowledge it.

Saturday morning when they were sleeping, I rolled its eighty-eight pounds down the front steps to the street. Ted hung onto the rail and walked to sit on the Amigo. He pressed the handle and took off at five miles per hour. *"Toot toot tootsie goodbye,"* he sang, waving in his now outdated wire glasses and denim cap. For the first time in years, I had to run to catch up to Ted.

"Hey mister!" a neighborhood kid called out. "Can I have a ride?" Ted stopped and took him aboard. It seemed a winner with all kids but ours.

Tacking, Ted could get the machine up the hill to the library. Breathing heavily as I ran, I rejoiced. Ted was free! The outdoors was his again!

When we got home the kids were still sleeping.

At supper, I lost my patience with Debbie over some unfinished homework. She burst into tears. She'd had a nightmare during her long sleep: looking out the junior high door at recess, she'd seen all the kids in the special education classes sitting on Amigos, riding in a circle around the soccer field. She stepped out to join them. The gym instructor warned her away: "This class is only for the defective!" Debbie opened her mouth to scream, "My father! My father!" and woke up.

"Come sit on my lap." Ted held out his arms and she touched down for a minute, but she was too old to sit on a lap for long. Her scene was now the school dance. Often I drove a carload of girls to a hall full of taped music and shy boys. Usually they laughed and talked on the way out but sat silent on the way home, tense with remembered moments of grief or thrill.

We ordered an Amigo anyway.

We must go on vacation together, the kids were growing so fast!

We opted for a weekend in Susan and Matt's vacant air-conditioned house in Boston. On a steamy day in July, Seth and I lifted Ted's new Amigo into the trunk, and after a night in Boston we lifted it out in front of the JFK library and set it on the wide plaza.

"That's repulsive!" Seth's eyes narrowed.

"I'm not going to look!" Debbie turned away.

"For Pete's sake!" I slammed the trunk. "It's hard enough for Daddy. Let's try to give him a little support." I could hear old family intonations in my voice.

Ted set his hat jauntily, stowed his cane, sat down, and puttered off. We walked behind him. You couldn't help but admire his courage. A breeze blew something into my contact lens. Inside the lobby, I ran to the ladies' room to fix it. Coming out, I saw Ted puttering across the shining floor toward me.

"You'd better help Seth." He puttered back and reached up

instead of his usual down to give the money to the cashier for the movie on JFK.

Seth stood with his forehead against the window.

"What's the matter?"

"If it's going to be like this, I want to jump out this window."

"Come on, shape up! It's time for the movie." In the worst of times, we fall back on the familiar.

We filed in to sit in a dark amphitheater. Charismatic Jack flickered before us in all his amazing youth. Seth wasn't watching: in the darkness tears rolled down his face. Perhaps John F. Kennedy was as timely to him as James K. Polk to us? Afterward we went for ice cream — double sundaes, the works, your basic infantile solution. We sat at our table for two hours and managed to lighten up. But they still wouldn't talk about the Amigo.

Ted didn't take it out anymore that summer.

How to defend the kids from Ted's frustrated outbursts? From my own frustrated outbursts? From my ineffectiveness? How to keep up the family foursome? Should I also try to do more healthy and normal things with the kids, leaving Ted out? He couldn't travel. He couldn't eat out. He seldom got to the movies. He went to bed early. He was often too hot or too cold. I couldn't think of much to do. Work had made me a dull girl. And fun takes money.

I rented out half the garage to a man with an antique car and filled an envelope with the thirty dollars. I wrote on it "Family Fun Money." It was for anything that at least two family members did together. The first month we went to the mall to the movies and had all the popcorn and sodas we wanted. But Seth chose the horror movie on screen B while the rest of us watched something calmer on screen A. Maybe he didn't want to be seen with his family? Thirty bucks wasn't enough for four to eat dinner out on, so we tried the all-you-can-eat Sunday brunch in town. That worked for three or four months. I walked Ted by the buffet and went back to fill his plate and mine. The kids got him seconds. After a while the kids said no. Rather sleep. Rather go with friends.

"They're too old for it," Ted suggested.

On the last day of one month the envelope was still full and I took a couple of dollars for breakfast with Thea, a new friend with whom I swam every morning at the YMCA. Debbie took a couple more for pizza with one of her friends. Seth took a few to play the dream machines at the mall. Ted didn't take any; he spent less on clothes, less on entertainment, and even less on doctors than we. He felt too responsible for the family's economic decline.

It was fear rather than fun that brought us together. Ted fell most often in the passageway between the yellow sunlit kitchen and the rosy wall-papered dining room. Usually he'd be carrying a dish. He would swerve, drop the dish, grab onto the wall. Then pause. Then he would fall gracefully, cleverly, not hitting his head, not cracking his skull. So fast that you couldn't move to catch him. Besides, he had the fall under control and if you moved in, you might throw off his carefully responding neurons. As soon as he lay still, he would assure us he was all right. Then he'd get up.

One autumn he cracked a rib falling onto the couch in his study. The next autumn he fell in the bedroom and heard a funny noise: his head hitting the floor. That afternoon, he fell against the television set. Against channel 8, as he put it. Chipped the base of a rib. Same as the year before. He began to use his cane indoors. I bought him a cordless, pocket-sized telephone, worried that he might fall and break a bone while I was at the office.

The choking was worse. At the table, Ted would gasp and struggle to breathe, bringing his hands to his throat. The first time, at a holiday, Mel and Doris and Susan and Matt and Susan's sons and all of us sat paralyzed. When Ted started to look a little blue, one of Susan's sons jumped up and gave him the Heimlich maneuver. Seth and I took a one-session course in it, to be ready.

As Debbie started high school and Seth his junior year, Susan suggested we meet with the principal and let him know some of the pressures on the kids. We did, asking the principal to advise the kids' teachers to encourage them a little. That first quarter Seth went out for the newspaper and Debbie made the honor roll. As things looked a little better on the youth front, other family members aged.

In Florida, Mel was having heart problems and some small seizures. Doris was lying awake to make sure he was breathing. They needed us.

In Connecticut, my mother had had two minuscule strokes,

leaving no damage although for a few weeks she had to "draw" her name instead of writing it. She needed us.

Whenever my mother was hospitalized, I took days off from my vacationless, benefitless, retirementless job to be with her. She needed more than I could give and she didn't dare ask for it. I wanted to give more; it just wasn't there to give. On the highway driving home from my renal failure to my sclerotic, I stopped once at the Mark Twain House in Hartford. I was simply too depleted to go on without something for myself.

It took me a long time to be able to feel the effect of the illness on the extended family. The old and the young lose attention and support. Instead of receiving from the flourishing generation in the middle, young and old alike must give and keep on giving.

"Worried about Nana and Grandpa?" I asked Debbie as she and I drove down to visit my mother one Sunday.

"That's certainly an understatement." She reached for the Kleenex as the tears ran down her cheeks. Debbie was learning how women keep families together from a rather ungraceful model.

My mother looked smaller but very much in charge of herself whenever we visited her in her small apartment in the big building with the three hundred seniors.

"How are you?" I would give her a hug: little, but steady on her feet.

"Fine." Although my mother had yearned to move to her continual care community, she was beginning to feel a little stuck there. She wanted long vacations with us, and trips to escape from the aged and dying — from the sudden loud arrival of ambulances. I gave a lot, but it was very little compared to what was needed.

We walked to her pleasant, restaurantlike dining room and found ourselves a table. An Amigo stood at the next table. Debbie seated herself so as not to see it.

In June, Mel and Doris drove north for a second opinion in Boston. Mel couldn't lift a gallon of milk. Mel couldn't get his shirt off over his head easily. It had been years since Ted could do either of these. We'd lost our sense of normalcy.

Mel looked pale. Things weren't going well. Maybe it was a less benign leukemia? Maybe the heart would go first? Maybe he didn't have as long as we'd thought.

He and Ted hugged goodbye on the porch. Susan and Matt would visit Florida in September. Susan's sons in the next months. Ted and I in January, when Ted could make the best use of and get the least damage from the sun.

At home, anger over the work load multiplied as I tried to switch more of it onto others. I felt like a prime mover trying to lever three sleeping elephants into place, or like a boss in a factory where sabotage had become the main activity.

"The grass is a foot high!"

"I didn't see it."

"Nobody put the garbage out!"

"You didn't tell me."

"Who left this in the refrigerator?"

"It's got mayonnaise on it."

"Why didn't you shut the attic windows?"

"It's not my job."

"Yes it is! See, it's right here on the list!"

It takes time to teach children to do chores they hate and time to make sure they do them. It takes energy and self-control and patience. I tried to be darling. I attempted charisma. I offered Jobs of Your Choice. We kept a rotating list. I analyzed the chores and found to my surprise how much supervisory work there is, how much time it takes to do research (for products, for workmen, for education) and to make decisions. I knew (see Appendix B, Hartmann) that most working mothers who hold 9-to-5 jobs come home to another thirty or thirty-five hours of housework. Homemakers with young children work a seventy-hour week. I was working from 8:00 to 4:00 five days a week and doing thirty hours more at home. Seth and Debbie and Ted split another seven or eight hours of housework. We all felt miffed and misused. I because I did the most. Seth because he handled the largest share of what I didn't do. Debbie because she preferred to be with friends. And Ted because he was embarrassed not to be able to do more. How to win in this chore game?

You tell me.

In August, Ted's left leg really seemed to be going. He saw the neurologist alone and the neurologist saw me alone in his small office with vertical blinds.

"How is he?" The neurologist took off his glasses.

"Depressed. Worried he's losing his left leg."

Ted returned from the examining room.

"Okay, I agree with you." The doctor turned to Ted. "It is time for you for think about Cytoxan. I wouldn't want to let you go down the tubes without a fight."

Driving home in the high-riding Buick, Ted was silent over the river so blue in the late summer light.

"What are you thinking?"

"What it would really be like to die. In, say, eight years, or ten. I mean really . . . die."

Hum of the bridge under wheels.

"What would it be like?"

"There are still books I want to write." He'd published four of his seventeen. He'd finished the history of Pericles, but it hadn't sold.

"Which ones?"

He named five or six, stretching his left leg out to rest it. "Maybe those last two are really the same book."

"Oh, Teddie."

Is that what it's like, then? You blend two books into one in order to get them done on time?

Instead of Cytoxan, Ted opted to go in for ACTH again. Perhaps that less harmful chemical would avert his right leg's decline. The nurses wheeled him into a room of semimoribunds sans teeth, sans everything. I could hear him making jokes faster and faster with nurses, with technicians — jokes, his own brand of life insurance.

His bedside phone rang and Susan reported that Mel had fallen in his hospital room in Florida. He'd been very shaken by it.

"Let's go down to Florida when you get out of here." I handed over the day's flowers, the day's newspaper. My father had died abruptly and I wanted to see Mel, wanted Ted to see Mel, wanted Mel to see Ted, not to mention the children.

We bought four tickets for late in September.

Mel worsened. Ted came home. We moved the tickets to earlier in September.

Two days before we were to fly, the phone rang. "My lovely Daddy is gone," Susan said.

We stood again in a quiet circle in the kitchen.

Seth had grown taller than Ted.

*   *   *

They brought Mel back on Delta. At the funeral, Ted slowly led the immediate family into a roomful of extended family and friends at the funeral service. Later, our children and Susan's walked beside the casket.

"That's the hardest thing I ever did," Seth said.

After a week of mourning in Boston, Seth's senior year marks fell slightly. Debbie's sank way down. Seth pulled out around Christmas and began to prepare his college applications. His SATs and achievements ran very high indeed, and he was a National Merit finalist. Surely he'd have colleges and offers of financial aid to choose from. I would pass his room full of jeans and tapes and record jackets and books and posters and maps and pencils and pennies and rumpled blankets and miles of electrical cord hung every which way for the stereo he'd saved up for and bought himself and think: next year it will be empty and still. How lonely we'd be!

Seth went out of communication writing his college applications. During Ronald Reagan's first term, benefits for the children of the disabled were ceased at eighteen instead of after college: Seth had to win financial aid. He began to seethe and shout. Was it just normal breaking away? Father and son nearly reached the breaking point. Once after a shouting tiff with Ted at the top of the back stairs, Seth explained why he was so enraged: "Because it's so humiliating! So embarrassing! To be shouted at by somebody you could knock down the stairs with a push!"

Debbie lay on the floor of her bedroom at midnight sobbing. "I don't want to be myself. I want to be anybody but myself!"

Report card: failing math, failing English.

"Go to sleep now. Try to sleep."

"I can't sleep!"

I debated Ted's Valium. No. Never. That was exactly what you feared with distraught teenagers — jumping out windows, gulping tranquilizers. Debbie's Highfield teachers began to suggest that perhaps we demanded too much. After all, we were writers. But back in Manhattan after her second eye operation when Debbie seemed to sag and fade, her teachers had wondered why we didn't expect more from her: she was as smart as her brother.

What to do? See the adjustment counselor. At the meeting, Debbie sat droopheaded, arms crossed in her lap, feet pointed in, eyes down. Her haircut completely veiled one eye. The counselor told us to set firmer limits, to make her study downstairs at the dining table without her radio. One of us should work along side her.

Ted didn't have the energy. I sat nightly from seven to ten for thirty arduous nights at a time when I felt Debbie should be breaking away from me — not to mention the hours added to my work week. Nothing she read went into her head. The best thing seemed to be when I read aloud to her. I read *Billy Budd* aloud.

"Read that sentence again!" She stopped me at the one lyrical sentence in Melville's nineteenth-century novella. "It's about the sea and it sounds just like the sea, isn't that neat?"

Flunked the quiz. Got the characters' names mixed up. Teacher didn't really believe she'd read *Billy Budd.*

Debbie skipped school and got caught. She left the house one night against our will. It no longer seemed like ordinary breaking away. Worried, we impressed her into psychotherapy.

Ted and I met with Dr. Rose. It was soothing to sit in the presence of a quiet pregnant worman wearing a French silk dress. How nice for Debbie; she needed tranquility.

"She's not self-destructive, but I can't get her to say one word about her father's illness," Dr. Rose reported. "What she talks about is friends. It may be that her feelings about the illness make a knot in her. It may be that she can't concentrate on schoolwork because of the knot. I'm not sure yet. Tell me, do you get depressed about the illness?" She looked at us. Ted didn't answer.

"Yes," I said.

"And how do you handle it?"

"I guess I get angry."

"And you, Ted?"

"Oh, no." He sat up straighter. "I just work and have my illness. I have no time for getting depressed."

One night in March we sat around the fireplace, Ted and Debbie and I. Seth was getting ready to go out in the car with friends. The Bookie group had expanded, and they went now to parties at the nearby college. I was reading Stephen Crane's "The Open Boat" to Debbie. In his chair not too near the fire,

Ted began to choke on a piece of candy. He was getting red in the face.

"Are you all right?" I said it calmly.

He stood up out of the chair, struggling to breathe.

"Are you all right?" I jumped up, shouting.

He shook his head no. Usually he nods yes. I got calmer instantly.

"Want the Heimlich?" I touched him gently.

He nodded yes, for the first time in years.

I got behind him and circled him with my arms; how small he was becoming. I found the right place and with my bent thumb drew him suddenly to me. You never know if you're really doing the Heimlich right. I tried it again. He was still gasping, growing blue.

"Seth!" I couldn't stand not having any help.

Seth came running down the stairs as I pressed a third time. He took over.

"Okay," Ted gasped, nodding.

Debbie appeared next to Ted, holding a glass of water.

"Wow, was I scared," I said a few minutes later, after Seth had gone back upstairs, after we three had sat down. We were supposed to talk about the fear, to get those feelings out in the open.

No reply.

"Were you scared?" I took up my book, adjusted the reading light.

No reply.

"How about you, Ted? Were you scared?"

"I was scared that time!" He came in on the message, although he was still coming down from his own terror. "It was scary all right!"

"Weren't you scared, Debbie?"

"Read," she instructed me, between her teeth. "Just read."

# Chapter 16
# How Devastating Illness Devastates the Family

Children are resilient; children bounce back. Do they? The children of a chronically ill parent grow up with the illness in their hearts. You can hear it in Barbara's statement.

She was thirteen in the 1950s when she began to notice something wrong about her father's arms. One swung differently from the other. Was it a brain tumor? She was sixteen when the last in a long string of doctors finally gave her mother the diagnosis. It was Parkinson's and the doctor said the patient mustn't know, it would devastate him. So Barbara's mother told Barbara instead.

My sister was away at college and didn't share the intimacy of the diagnosis. I became my mother's confidante. We whispered together. I became a parent to my father and he became like a child to me. I felt tremendous protectiveness for both my parents. My father's being sick affected me a lot. It didn't allow me the normal range of disappointments and hostilities. It's made me compassionate, but it imposed a very heavy burden on me as a child.

Chronic illness brings chronic anger. I felt annoyed from both my father's point of view and my own. I felt his shame, the humiliation he shouldn't have felt but did, when he couldn't get up and talk in front of a group. He felt compromised by the illness and I felt compromised for him. From my own point of view, I felt the classic *Why did this have to happen to me?* It wasn't until I experienced a pregnancy during which I had to lie in bed for seven months — three in a hospital — that I understood how my father must have felt. I was forced to lie there, to be totally dependent on other people. That's the closest I ever felt to my father.

He was very stoic. He took it in what you'd call a very British manner. He suffered a devastating, deteriorating illness from age forty-seven to age seventy-three and never complained. I wish he had screamed and yelled and raged. We would have felt closer to him. It would have validated some of our own frustration and anger, my mother's and mine. I could have reached out to him. It was hard to do that when he wouldn't talk about it. I felt that I was part of his life and not part of it.

Grown up, I have tried to follow my father's example of courage and endurance. I didn't allow myself to show grief over my sorrows — and by comparison, nothing in my life matches up. My own emotions seem to pale, become less valid.

When you're young you have to have a time of innocence. I knew from thirteen that I was no longer protected, and I didn't understand why I shouldn't be. I wish I'd had a greater sense of optimistic future. I missed that unlimited, unbounded future that kids and young people need. We were always concerned about money. My mother explained from the moment of the diagnosis that I'd have to work while I was a college, and I did, all the time. I never had that adolescent headiness, that sense of the world belonging to me.

I can remember meeting my future in-laws, how vigorous and healthy they looked! I felt very protected. They were big, sturdy people. My own children are seven and eight now, and it's always given me great joy to see my husband throw them in the air. My family has a much greater feel of optimism, more enthusiasm, more sense of the future, though I have become very health conscious. I never say, "We're all healthy." I say, "This year everyone's all right."

It's hard for a child watching an extraordinary battle for survival to say she wants to go to the movies. I knew how hard it was on my parents. There is so much guilt for the child.

Barbara tried. Her mother tried. Her father tried. It isn't easy.

Child therapist Anita Glicken, M.S.W., who teaches at the Child Health Associate Program in the medical school at the

University of Colorado, also knows from the inside how hard it is. Her mother got cancer when Anita was five and had it for five years, although she seldom discussed it. People didn't talk about cancer in the 1950s and 1960s. Anita's mother checked in and out of the hospital as if every mother did that. Even Anita's teenaged siblings didn't discuss it. When Anita was ten, her mother died.

> From then on, it was chronic loss. I felt alienated from my father. I felt angry and hostile because my father was safe, he hadn't died. You vent your frustration wherever you feel safest and least guilty. So the well parent may get the most attack. Not until adulthood did I have a decent relationship with my father.
>
> And it's never gone — the sense that I might get sick. That's much more of an everyday reality than it is for other people.

Glicken lists the following as emotions and responses parents can expect from their children if one parent is chronically ill. Her list reads like our own Chronic Emotions but may be imagined now from the child's point of view. Glicken describes each response.

*Denial.* A long-term refusal to face the problem.

*Helplessness.* A real and continued feeling of inadequacy and disorganization. If a child's needs are not met consistently, he or she may learn to feel inadequate.

*Guilt.* A child may have both good and bad wishes about a parent. Then, if the parent gets sick, the child feels responsible because of bad wishes. This process peaks around age five, yet the connection between desire, behavior, and outcome never goes completely away: it remains as the Why Me response.

*Chronic Anger.* This is typically directed not only at the sick parent but at everybody else — for not meeting the child's needs.

*Jealousy.* It's very easy for a child to feel that someone is taking all the attention — even if the child is getting attention.

*Embarrassment and Shame.* This is a developmental issue for a child. It's hard to master shame if you feel you have something to be ashamed of. Adolescents may be embarrassed to have a relative who looks different. These issues must be dealt with over and over as the child develops.

*Ambivalence.* There's a real desire to help and also a real anger and revulsion. Why can't you be normal? Ambivalence makes everything the child has to master harder: independence, attachment, separation. For instance, if a child feels so very needed at home, he or she can't separate easily.

*Chronic Grief.* There's a real bereavement over the loss of the dreams of the family that was to be. Why can't we be like the Cosbys? Like Ozzie and Harriet? There's a real recognition at a much earlier age than usual that life may not be happy.

*Chronic Depression.* The potential is there for children to be very withdrawn and isolated.

"A parent knows a child better than anybody else," Glicken points out. "If you sense something amiss, consider whether it is or isn't connected to the sickness. There might be other bothersome things — school, peers, identity problems, vocation issues, role models."

What to do if children seem to be in trouble? Glicken recommends encouraging them to become involved with other adults — the parents (ones you approve of) of their friends or adults found in religious groups. Religion can be very helpful. "A child can say, 'God's doing it and He has His reasons.' " This, Glicken reasons, takes the blame off the child. But religion can be troubling if the child wonders why God is punishing his parents and himself so much. " 'Are Mommy and Daddy being bad in some way I don't know about?' And in that case, 'Will I get sick? Will it happen to me?' "

If a child is in real trouble and you see no solution, try a counselor — if the child is willing. "But don't jump the gun," Glicken warns, "it may just be adolescence."

"Set limits," she urges. "With chronic illness, there's a tendency for parents not to push kids. They figure enough has been asked of the child already."

"One advantage of chronic illness," Glicken adds, "is that you get time to go over things with children." It may be hard for parents to say just what they're feeling, and children often pick up on the exact unspoken feeling and express it: "How come you didn't take care of Daddy so this wouldn't happen?" That would be very hard for a woman to deal with at the moment she might be having the same thought. There's plenty of time. Deal with things when you're able.

Glicken concludes: "Watch for the child's needs. If a child loses her toy, that's a big issue. It may be that her father can't walk, but the parent has to make the child feel that the lost toy is the most important thing right then. The parent has to make the child feel that his problems or needs are as important as the needs of the sick parent. As grown-ups, these children look back and wonder how they could have felt that their needs were equal. But they learn to sort out as they grow only if their needs were met as children. The parent becomes the model of how to deal with things, and if the parents accept the illness and incorporate it into their lives, the children will."

In psychological testing of the children of families where one parent had MS, David Rintell, Ed.D, of the Framingham (Massachusetts) Youth Guidance Center, found them to be a bit sad, a bit anxious, and slightly pseudomature, but not neurotic. "This is a healthy response," Dr. Rintell points out, "because it's realistic."

He found a mitigating circumstance. "The more the family shares tasks and the more the sick parent does in the home, and the more flexible the mother and father are about sex role division of labor, the better it is for their children." In his study (see Appendix B), Dr. Rintell discerned that the more decision making the sick parent held onto, the better it was for the children's sense of themselves. He observed that it was harder for men to be flexible about role change than women and that in households where the woman was sick, adaptation appeared to go more smoothly.

In talks with his subjects, Dr. Rintell came frequently upon anger. "If the sick parent is angry, he may not be angry at the kids but they don't know that. He may be a geyser. He may explode. The kids run away. They can get burnt by the hot water. The farther they get, the safer they feel. But anger doesn't kill you. It's the growing distance between a child and an angry parent that's the problem. Anger drives a wedge of distance. If there is too much distance, it's like the loss of a parent. And that's the real problem."

Dr. Rintell offers modifications to the three traditional danger signs in children — a drop in schoolwork, rebelliousness, and depression. In his work at the center, he has found a subgroup of kids who do well in school no matter how they may be suffering. They may go home to such dire things as sexual abuse while their grade point averages never slip below 4. "School is the only part of their lives that goes well." Similarly, a child may be depressed without displaying either disturbances in eating and sleeping (too much, too little) or rebelliousness against rules. Some kids show depression simply by tuning out. "It's the same as when you try to handle an upset by not feeling it; it's a denial. A child who speaks only about the problem or who never can speak of it is in trouble. It's tricky. A lot of teenagers tune out anyway. But if you work with children, you know this kind of thing when you see it."

What about the parents of the sick spouse? Of the well spouse? What about siblings? Nephews? Nieces? Aunts? Uncles? The whole family suffers the shock and loss of the acute emotions. Over the years some family members move toward the chronic emotions. Notice the spread of response through Ted's family and mine when asked, nine years later, how his MS had affected them.

Ted's mother: "I can't answer. It's too close to my heart. It doesn't matter how old the child is, it hurts." (What sorrow is greater than terrible damage to one's child? It puts the spouse experience into perspective.)

His sister: "At first I was so anxious. I can get pretty depressed if I allow myself to think about it in negative ways. I feel guilty that we're traveling and enjoying our leisure and you two find that almost impossible. I wish I could do more."

Her husband: "I feel sadness and concern for Susan and the family. The four of us do fewer things together. The illness moves in on the person so inevitably that you feel a sense of desperateness because you can't change its course — the person becomes almost a drama to be watched."

A nephew: "It has brought enduring and increasing sorrow. It's painful to watch Uncle Ted's deterioration and his struggle to maintain his dignity."

A nephew: "It made me angry and sad, and guilty that I'm healthy and the world is not. If there's a genetic component, what are the chances that I'll get it or my brothers? Cousins?"

A nephew: "I was going off to college when I heard and it was the last big nail in the 'unfair coffin.' When Grandpa got throat cancer it was because he smoked cigars but Uncle Ted hadn't done anything to get MS. When the family gets together people say 'Did you hear what Matt is doing? Did you hear what Seth is doing? Did you hear what So-and-So is doing? Did you hear how Ted *is*?' It's as if nothing he does now matters. And, I can't believe I'm saying this, but the whole thing gets boring."

My mother: "I can't imagine how it could be worse for Ted. It's sad to see you work so hard. You have dreams for your children. I had dreams for you."

My brother: "Ted handles the steady cruelty of it very well. My concern is for you and Seth and Debbie. It seems, in some strange way, that the disease has affected you three more than Ted. I feel I should help more, but there doesn't seem that much an individual can do. I worry about how you will manage if he can't walk."

A niece: "I was thirteen when I heard and it was scary to visit because we didn't visit very often and it was always shocking. Uncle Ted has the kind of courage they don't give out medals for. I learned very young that good and bad are irrelevant, that believing in God is no insurance, that good doesn't always win."

Clearly these responses run the gamut from the acute to the chronic emotions, depending upon age, frequency of contact, and relationship. The family feels what you feel, with different emphases and intensities. There is little the well spouse can do to alleviate the suffering of the extended family, except to give honest reports and to learn to take help gracefully. All our energy is needed for the home.

How does family giving affect us? Lots. It's essential. Some families offer only a bravura cheerleading for the sick person; others provide vital practical aid for all. You can hear the difference between the presence and absence of family support in the following two accounts.

In Maine, Jerilyn was forty when diabetes first blinded her. Her family and her husband's family lived nearby. Steve says:

> Jerilyn's parents came during the day, if Jerilyn was down. Once after an operation when she was in bed for three months, they brought meals over and picked up the kids at school. They'd come and visit, just be there for her. My mother made us meals when Jerilyn had her eye operations. All that help made me feel good, made me feel that the problem wasn't mine alone.
>
> I become more involved with our youngest child. Abby started school and I would make more of her at school plays, doubling my comments. "Gee, you looked really pretty tonight," or "you did very well." I played with her at night, too, I read to her — more so than I'd done with the other two.
>
> My son was very good about it. It was killing him that Jerilyn

couldn't see. He's very close to her. He would tease her, pick on her, get her to laugh, making jokes about being blind. If she didn't hear something he'd say, "God, Mom, it's bad enough you're blind, you going to lose your hearing now?" She'd laugh. That was his way of handling it. He liked to mow the lawn. What's my secret? You've got to buy a tractor! He loves to sit up there and mow.

My older daughter, Scotty, is like a mother hen. She tried very, very hard. I couldn't have gotten by without her help. I think she felt that she would have to spend the rest of her life taking care of the family. This did change when Jerilyn learned to take care of the house even though she was blind. When Scotty got married, Jerilyn couldn't really see Scotty coming down the aisle. But we enjoyed ourselves immensely, anyway.

I don't know if the kids have suffered. They had more responsibility. They had to help out with housework, picking up their rooms. They did it very willingly. They were happy to do it. They all realize that life isn't peaches and cream. Problems come up in life. They've learned to stick together to help one another out.

We all went swimming twice a week and cross-country skiing every weekend. We would go skiing when Jerilyn was blind — someone in front of her and someone in back. We'd yell out "duck your head," or "going down a slope," or "take a right hand turn." We were together as a family. We've always been very close as a family and we still are.

It wasn't only family that helped Steve. Again, the severity of illness matters. Jerilyn could function: she learned to do all her housekeeping without sight and she continued to manage her diabetes strictly. She knew exactly what was going on, and she and Steve remained a close team — as we'll see further in chapter 18. A close pair increases the likelihood of a close family.

Things were different for Alix, who had little help from a widely scattered extended family. Indeed, she had opposition. Harvey's illness affected his thinking, and his parents refused to believe this for years. Again, the particular illness matters. When thinking is modified, the well spouse becomes far more alone in the marriage and the children basically bereaved. Alix describes the arduous process by which her husband went, as she put it, subtly mad, and how this affected her and each of their children differently.

We moved to Maryland in 1971 because Harvey wanted to get out of academic medicine and do a little something more for mankind. We'd adopted four children in Manhattan and we had a wonderful life there, but Harvey had a hankering to practice medicine in a rural area and so we came here. For a couple of years things were fine. Then in the summer of 1973 Harvey's brother got married and we were driving back late at night from Pittsburgh in the station wagon. Dickie was three, so Tanya would have been five and the older ones seven and nine. Tanya traveled very well, but it was late at night and she had to pee. She asked Harvey to stop by the side of the road. He said no, she should wait till she got home. "Just pull over to the side of the road," I said, "and let her out." But he wouldn't. I couldn't believe it. It wasn't like him. Tanya's a no-sweat child, not a complainer. I turned around to see this little girl standing up behind the front seat silently with tears rolling down her face. I asked again. He wouldn't stop. Swearing is not my thing, but I said, "How can you be such a son-of-a-bitch!" It seemed so cruel and unexplained. I figured maybe he was in a foul mood because of the drive late at night.

About a year later, Tanya was crossing the kitchen. Harvey said something to her and when she didn't answer, he took her by the shoulders and pushed her into the cabinet. She cried. Harvey never exploded with the children. I was the short-tempered parent. Harvey never minded playing Candyland 950 times. I'm the one that kicks the cat if the washing machine and septic system break on the same day.

That winter, Harvey went to a smoking clinic and gave it up. He seemed depressed and tired all the time. He said that was normal for giving up smoking. He became impotent. He got the flu. It was a funny kind of flu that left him feeling as if his fingers had been in ice water. He had difficulty buttoning his shirt collar. I would come home and find him sleeping at 2:30 in the afternoon.

I worked at the hospital where he practiced, and one day a colleague took me aside to ask if Harvey were depressed. The cardiologists reread all the EKGs at night and they'd picked up some sloppiness in Harvey's readings. He was usually so precise.

The symptoms continued. In the spring of 1976 we went to a neurologist about the tingling. The neurologist did a spinal and told Harvey he might have MS, but there were no clinical signs. He sent Harvey to an internist, who found a thyroid problem. (When you're a doctor, your colleagues identify with you and are afraid to find anything seriously wrong with you.) He needed a thyroid supplement. No wonder he was depressed! No wonder he was tired!

Six weeks of thyroid medicine didn't help. He remained irritable and irascible and he blamed it on me. It was my fault because I didn't like Maryland. I believed it. I must be setting him off. I shouldn't be grumpy.

Harvey's secretary said he was falling asleep at his desk. His neurologist said I was impatient about his recovery. His mother told me I shouldn't be working with four small children at home. A friend corroborated my sense that Harvey was depressed and told me I should get him to a psychiatrist even though he didn't want to go. One night I walked into the den and told Harvey that either he'd see a psychiatrist or I would leave with the children.

He went to the psychiatrist, who put him on six weeks of antidepressants for what he called a typical mid-life crisis. New Year's Eve when we took the children skiing, Harvey couldn't keep his balance. He tried a second course of drugs. He tried a third.

Harvey remained aggressive and hostile. He'd tell the children, "Your mother is going to commit suicide." He would attempt to choke me. I knew that if I gave him a shove, he'd lose his balance and fall. I never shoved him. He'd come in covered with mud from rototilling the garden and get into bed without a shower. He was incontinent and unshaven and disheveled.

By summer I was getting hysterical. Harvey's psychiatrist said I wasn't handling Harvey's depression supportively. I should see a psychiatrist. In my first session, the psychiatrist asked me to describe the problem. At the end of fifty minutes, he said, "You have just described a case of organic brain syndrome." He handed me a piece of paper. "Go back and ask them to do these tests."

The CAT scan found moth holes in the part of the brain that controls emotions. He lost his job and kept on degenerating slowly. Today he is institutionalized. He doesn't blink an eye.

He doesn't speak. He doesn't recognize me. He doesn't recognize the children.

Bob is twenty-three and William twenty-one and Tanya nineteen and Dick seventeen. Only now am I hearing their pain. For years, Bob has told me I ruined his life. He's angry, angry that he had to step into his father's shoes and be responsible. Angry that he had no childhood. That he had to be serious. Sometimes I get impatient and sometimes I just feel sorry for him. I say, "Bob, you were born serious. You were a serious baby. You played chess when you were five." He tells me I don't understand the horror of having Dad around.

William was always dreamy and musical. He's had some trouble with drugs and alcohol — his school therapist didn't even pick up on the fact that he was smoking pot. He says that growing up was horrendously painful. He felt I had so much pain that he couldn't burden me with anything else. When Harvey stopped working, I went back to graduate school at night while holding a full-time job and driving four kids to four schools. From my point of view, I kept it all together. From their point of view, I'd race out the door in the morning and come back to make supper and drive back into the city to school. They felt there wasn't any energy and time for them. They had to make their pickups on the fly. They had to be standing at the front gate of school at 5:16 or whatever. They minded that split-second scheduling. If they were off schedule, I'd be irascible. And of course I was in a state of high anxiety. What would I find at the end of the ride home? Would Harvey be lying at the bottom of the stairs? Or wedged in the shower? Or getting ready to chase Dick with a chair? Maybe it would just be a note from my mother-in-law telling me there was nothing wrong with Harvey.

Tanya was born smiling and she continues to smile. She's like me, and maybe it's good for her and maybe it isn't. I may have a very tough exterior, but that's not all of me. I felt I couldn't let one tear out or I'd be like the wicked witch of Oz and melt and disappear. The kids would have lost their last parent and been terrified.

When Dick developed a tic in third or fourth grade, I whisked him off to be tutored and to see a psychiatrist. Now Dick can speak of the illness the easiest of any of them. Tremendous attention went to this child because his pain was clearly visible.

Last year he visited Harvey with me. He announced that he was never going to visit again.

We had to separate our assets and start divorce proceedings so I could manage the nursing home without losing the house, but I still feel married. I visit twice a year. There's still no diagnosis. The top candidate is a slow, exotic virus picked up during his stint in the Peace Corps. Sometimes it feels as if the saddest thing is that Harvey and I never got to talk about what was happening to him and to the kids.

Send this woman roses.

————◄◉►————

## HOW ARE THE KIDS?

Ideally, children need healthy, energetic, warm, involved parents. Whatever deviates from this makes a lack. Children handle the lacks differently. Some think they're sick themselves. Some find surrogate parents. Some leave home too early or too late. Some become more isolated and depressed, some rebellious. We watch. As Kathy in Georgia watches:

> I see the scars and joys of normal childhood, but I also see the pain and growth that come from having a disabled daddy. At first with my son it was "Why my daddy?" But gradually he's come to see that other children don't have perfect families either. Other kids may have no dad or mom, or parents who fight and drink. He talks with me often. He is my sounding board. He's done a lot of growing and has taken on many responsibilities around the house. My only hope is that he doesn't grow up too fast. I make sure I allow for his play time and keep remembering he's only ten!
>
> My daughter at seven barely remembers piggyback rides from Dad. She loves and hugs her dad to the point where she'll climb on the arm of his chair or hang on to the side rail of his bed. She is not the open talker her brother is, and I wonder how much worry and pain she carries around.

Do look for signs of change: trouble at school, breaking the rules, eating or sleeping problems, drugs.

Do speak about how life and the future have changed.

Do assure young children that the illness is not their fault.

Do emphasize that life will go on.

Do notice if one child pushes too hard to fill parental shoes — this is apt to be the first child or the child of the same sex as the sick parent.

Do work to reestablish contact between the sick parent and the children. If there is no personality change from cerebral damage, the whole group reintegrates. If you have relied on a certain child through the opening crisis, be conscious of letting go and reestablishing family unity.

Do watch for when you must protect children and for when you mustn't intrude on the integrity of the sick parent.

Do talk. Listen to each other. You don't have to agree.

Do encourage the sick person to say how hard things are, how hard he's trying. Then the well people may speak.

Do try to meet the immediate needs of children — even if the larger issues are out of control.

Do go for family therapy if you think even one member is depressed, isolated, or stuck in a rut. That person may be suffering for all of you. Try a few visits and then stop and evaluate to see if you're getting anything from it.

Do assure the child (if it's true) that the illness isn't hereditary.

Do have fun! After midteens, it's too late to expect children to want to start a lot of family activities that haven't already proven themselves to be fun.

Do ask friends to take a child hiking or bowling or swimming. Ask friends to be like godparents to a child. Ask them to tell the kids they look terrific, healthy.

Don't blame everything on the illness.

# Chapter 17
# *What's Left of the Two of Us?*

The June that Seth graduated from high school, we celebrated our twentieth wedding anniversary at Ted's favorite restaurant, the one with the flowers and the silver coffee pots. He's been there three times. Twenty years before we'd spent a weekend on Fire Island, eating grilled cheese sandwiches and looking forward to children, books, and walking together over Ireland and Greece.

"Happy anniversary." With his left hand, Ted raised his glass of wine a token quarter inch. He took a token sip. Wine destroys what balance he has left. His eyes lightened. "It's bound to be a richer and a better year!"

"How come?" I raised my glass.

"Because we've already had poorer and worse and in sickness."

We smiled.

I love Ted. He loves me. We are friends who have known each other twenty-one years. We are loyal to each other. I wouldn't want it to end, although I dread living like this, and worse, for the rest of my life. What's left of us?

Not our mutual independence. Ted grows more and more dependent physically, emotionally, and even financially. The war without roses prickles, there is resentment at the illness that can never be shed. We're bored with the degeneration that

224

keeps us living on an emotional and social subsistence level. Knowing or verbalizing this doesn't particularly help. The illness is still here, still winning.

When the kids were little, we used to play a board game called Chutes and Ladders. Now Ted and I play it in life. A chute leads right down under our dining room, under our bedroom, under our front yard. I don't think of it as a chute, but as a downward ladder. That's because of something I read in an MS newsletter years back. If I could find it, I'd certainly ascribe it to its wise originator, a psychiatrist with MS. He said that having this disease is like going down a ladder. He said forget the inspirational books. You don't have to be happy and cheerful all the time. You have to grieve. You have to grieve on each rung of the ladder down. You grieve when you lose walking. You grieve when you lose vision. And so forth. You go down step by step. It's natural, it's normal, it's right to grieve these losses. However, you do find footing on each rung as you descend. You do learn to balance again on each rung. There comes a time on each rung when you feel a little better, feel a little more in control, feel a little more mastery. And then you do down another rung.

Here's how we walked to the car the summer Seth graduated. First, across the porch, Ted's left leg moving somewhat normally and his left hand using the cane. His right leg dragged unbent from backward to forward. With his right hand up to his chest, his shoulders rode at an uneven height. His right knee threatened to buckle at any time. Would it support him on this step? On the next? I took his hand as he started down the stairs. His hand was cold and didn't grasp mine but rested in it, not exactly like a child's, more like an old person's hand — yet not so strong. We cleared the downgrade of the stairs. I slowed my pace to match Ted's. It was difficult even for me, whose muscles obey her nerves, to balance at that very delayed pace. We started across the tarred walk to the driveway. He could relax now. He said, "What are you walking so fast for?"

I was free of the illness in my own body: the balance I had to strike was not in my body but in my marriage with Ted. I hate being Mama. I hate being the rock. Wasn't I born a butterfly? The more I take over the things Ted needs me to do, the more he takes control of me. Yet if I put my major emphasis on maintaining some well life with friends — brief flights to the

YMCA pool, to lunches — I begin to feel too separated from Ted, and if I resolve to focus more on Ted, I feel stifled and restless at home.

I think often of a woman who came up to me after a support group I'd visited. Her husband had been sick and in pain for forty-five years. "You can have a normal life," she assured me. "All you have to do is stop doing whatever your husband can't do. When my husband stopped swimming, I stopped swimming. When he stopped bowling, I stopped bowling. We took up camping. You find new things to replace the old. He couldn't play baseball with our kids, but those kids both played a crackerjack game of chess by the time they were five. When he stopped working, he began to fall. He broke an arm. He broke a leg. He broke his neck. The doctor said, 'You've got to hire somebody to stay with him and keep him down or you've got to quit your work and be with him." So I quit work. I hated that. I don't think he has any idea how much I hated quitting work. I loved my job. I hated quitting, but I don't have any regrets — do you understand what I mean? I have no regrets. I wouldn't want him to know how much I hated quitting. It would be too hard for him."

To me that's not a normal life.

Sometimes I make an effort to bring a *New York Times* or a flower home to Ted. I enter the kitchen full of good cheer and put the flower in a vase only to hear him making his slow way down the back stairs, only to have him swallow his words so I can't hear them, only to find myself switching to Red Alert. The flower's tender sentiments vaporize.

That's it for tonight, folks.

I'm impatient.

My return to the house is usually the day's big social moment for Ted. I'm the amusement. I'm the outside world. I'm the breath of discovery. And here she is, already impatient. He proceeds, because he is a grown-up and not easily flattened.

"Let me read you something." He takes a small book from his pocket.

Oh, I should be grateful he isn't morose. I should laugh and smile. But that particular night the phone was ringing and Debbie wasn't home to answer it and Seth was working evenings as a telephone solicitor and I couldn't find the recipe for the new pasta. It was a friend for Debbie and I told him to call back at six. Something fell off the herb shelf. There was sugar crunching under my feet.

"Pretty good, isn't it?" Ted finished and looked up from the rocker.

I hadn't heard a word.

"Hmmm."

Then he was hurt. He got up to pour himself a drink of cranberry juice. He got the jar out okay. He carried it to the table. I curtailed my movements, holding the pot full of water longer than is comfortable for my aging elbow. Smile. Finally set it on the burner. Whew. Relief. He was standing in front of the silverware drawer. Careful. Wait. I got out the onions instead. Gosh but I was tired. Only three or four hours of sleep in the night, despite the newly arranged twin beds. Managed a twenty-minute nap on the office floor.

"Damn it!" he shouted. "You told me you were going to get a new bottle opener!"

A new bottle opener was item 87 on my list of essential do-it-nows.

"I'll get it for you," I said, meaning both the opener and this particular cap.

He shoved it at me, threw the rubber opener after it.

I got the cap off. New jar. Too full. Too heavy. Should I ask? No. Yes. "Do you want me to pour it?"

"No! I will!"

Ah, both mad.

Susan and Matt sit at the dining table with the maps of their trip to the British Isles spread out.

"In this town we're staying at the Hermes Hotel." Susan points to a spot on the map.

"They used to call it the Herpes," Ted suggested. "But they changed the name instead of the sheets."

We're jealous of their trip; they're guilty about going.

Our old joy in exploration has gone. The number of things we like to do that we can do together shrinks continually. Riding around the countryside, exploring old towns or old buildings, visiting bookstores or libraries, slipping out for a glass of wine, even going to the movies, are all lost to us. Long before them went biking or hiking or canoeing or simply walking around the block together on a summer evening. We can sit on the porch. We can read. We can have people over (work) and we can go to their houses (that's it!).

Sometimes, watching "Masterpiece Theatre" in our afghans, it seems that we have only aged before our time. And, in a way, that's exactly what's so painful about chronic illness — it's premature aging. I'm glad to have aged with someone who makes me laugh. Someone who surprises me with tidbits at supper. Someone who's loyal. I can't imagine living with a healthy man who returns every evening with briefcase and tennis racquet but who doesn't really care to know what Seth is doing, or Debbie. Who doesn't remember the mornings they were born. Who didn't read Classic Comics in Greek. Or tell me he'd discovered the first time we met for a romantic lunch, as he leaned across the table to take my hand by the wavering candle, that — upon examination of my wrist and arm — I had the measles.

"You make a lousy patient," he informed me in the days when he could walk and carry trays and sit upon the bed beside me.

He does better at it than I would.

I've had to separate in some ways, and it sometimes feels as if I'm not really married. I've begun to dream that I'm back in college with everyone except me getting married. Sometimes it's so painful to watch Ted get weaker that I don't watch.

We've polarized into optimistic and pessimistic. Ted makes jokes about life's little problems; I notice that the furnace isn't running. We've polarized into isolated and social. Sometimes I'm too tired to enjoy the parties I give to bring people into the house, but I'm afraid to stop. And we've polarized into care giver and care receiver. Ted does take care of me, too, though. Once in a while when I can't sleep and he's not trying to fade out with a fresh Valium, he tells me stories of Belle Indifference, an imaginary heroine who dances her nights away. If Paris falls, she dances; if Brazil sinks, she dances; if the waters in Venice rise, she dances. If . . .

Not the full traditional male and female remains — we find our place within what's left. The seasons come and go. Ice on the twigs, forsythia in April and the budding branches. One May was so beautiful that I thought continually of naked men, well men, powerful of thigh — they had no faces. Ted somehow perceived it and made more of it than was there. I sat on his bed to say goodbye before going off to my morning swim, but his eyes were narrow and dark.

"You've got something going with Art." He named a neighbor.

"That's crazy!"

I did fantasize. Who doesn't? I did flirt. Who doesn't? But I had remained faithful to Ted and I wanted some credit for it. I told him so. "And if I were in you shoes," I concluded, "I'd have given you free rein, anyway. Just so long as you didn't tell me about it."

"Well, not me," he replied. "I'll never do that. And if I catch you with someone, I'll kill him. The MS is a blow for both of us, man and wife. I have to accept it. You have to accept it, too."

On my way downstairs I realized he'd overlooked an essential point: although he could never escape the illness, I could. I could walk out the front door any morning of my life and not come back. When I didn't, I was opting for MS, opting for what he'd quit in a flash if he could. And my reward for this was to be falsely accused?

Why Art? The preceding weekend, I'd clipped branches and then stepped into the garage onto an iron rake left tines-out and it slammed me in the face. Broken tooth? No. Split lip, blood, swelling, pain. No one in my family noticed it all evening. The next day Art walked by as Ted and I were getting into the car.

"What happened to your lip?" Art said. I showed it to him.

"Goodbye, trees." Ted settled into the passenger seat and Debbie into the back. "Next time you see me, I'll be dancing!"

Ted opted for chemotherapy — walk more now, endure fewer of the vegetable years later.

"Daddy may not look any different when he comes back," I hurriedly and hatefully warned Debbie. Don't expect too much, the leaflet on Cyclophosphamide had urged — this was Cytoxan with a longer name. You could be very disappointed. You could get very depressed.

"Look, Maggie, I have to psyche myself up!"

"I know, I know."

The drug's threat of possible leukemia in ten years had mellowed (or so we thought, somewhat mistakenly) to possible kidney trouble in twenty years — that's progress for you. What scared Ted the most was that the dirty drug might not work for him. That he'd end up in the 30 pecent of nonresponsives. That he wouldn't make the 70 percent of responsives who by using the drug delayed going from one cane to two or from two canes to the wheelchair. That he'd really lose his hair this time. That it had come to this.

Don't hit the tree. Buckle up for the highway. How will I navigate Boston's one-way streets? Find the Boston Museum School and the Massachusetts College of Art for Debbie's tours? Is the mayonnaise in the sandwiches turning? At least I didn't have to worry about the car falling apart: we had inherited Mel's Volvo.

"Move the lunch basket out of the sun, Debbie."

"No," Ted said, at some chance remark of mine.

"No," I said at one of his.

No.

No.

No.

That's how scared we were.

At two o'clock we dropped Ted off at the door of the Brigham and Women's Hospital and went to park. In the lobby everyone was walking fast and Ted was gone.

"An aide must have taken Daddy off in a wheelchair."

"Everybody walks so fast in Boston." Debbie was my height now, her beautiful black hair cut to half an inch most of the way around. She dressed in what appeared to her parents to be an assortment of underclothes. In actuality, she arranged herself rather superbly and even conservatively in the newest fashion.

Ted was wearing a shirt over his pajamas, determined to stay uninfantilized. Doris, without Mel, sat on his bed.

"Your hair doesn't fall out until after a few weeks," the man in the next bed explained. He was a repeater. "And sometimes it grows back curly."

"Curly! I can't wait."

"If it takes a couple of weeks, I may not be bald when we take Seth to college."

Seth had won a large scholarship and was due to start college in two weeks, back in his old home, New York.

*     *     *

"There are so many women doctors now." I tried to encapsulate some history for Debbie in the elevator. "Twenty years ago you seldom saw women doctors."

"Can we stop off at three? To see the babies?"

So we stood in front of them, one pink, one brown.

"Aren't they terrific!" I put my arm around her. What terrible illnesses might lurk in those sleeping packages of DNA?

With his eyes closed, Ted could touch his nose with his finger for the first time in years.

"Worth losing my hair to find my nose." He sat up in pajamas.

He could shake hands with his right hand. He could pick up the phone with his right hand and call Seth on his eighteenth birthday.

But don't get excited, the doctors said. It might not be the Cyclophosphamide. It might just be the preparatory ACTH.

"I know your first duty is to your husband," my mother said wistfully over Ted's bedside phone. "I know I shouldn't expect you to come down and take me into the hospital."

"He's doing wonderfully," Susan said into the phone by my mother's bedside in New Haven. "His voice is stronger. They're giving him voice therapy. We have to tell him to quiet down!" But don't get excited. It might be nothing.

He could walk better.

He had more energy.

But don't.

"Stand together, guys. I've got to get used to the heights." They stood before me by the refrigerator where the photograph of two grown boys had once been taped. "He's really taller. He's a lot taller!"

"That's only because he's wearing socks!" Ted said, in his bare feet. The doctors at the Brigham had taken him off his amphetamine and he seemed less angry.

"My socks have got holes in them!" Seth countered. How happy they looked, the one to be taller, the other to be shorter.

"I'm not even bald," Ted rejoiced the next day, as we sat on a wall and watched the college freshmen guiding their parents through hundreds of blue balloons hanging over the campus in

Manhattan. Seth was unloading his things from the car, refusing aid from his mother. He looked tall and lean in his dirty I-don't-care tee shirt, carrying in his stereo. Ted sat and fingered the denim cap in his lap. He'd brought it along, in case.

At home, Seth's room was empty and still, and the first night I felt sad. The next morning I woke happy: Seth was exploring the great world. He'd made it out with who knew what damage, but he'd made it.

What's left? Ted. Me. Ted and me. To be known by someone over many years provides a basic "I am" of identity essential to sanity. We trust and respect each other just as we did when we married, only now it has been tested. The marriage remains; the marriage changes; the marriage remains.

In the kitchen that Labor Day when Jane and Patrick were visiting, Ted stumbled and I reached out to steady him.

"I saw what passed between you," Jane told me later. "If I'd had that in my marriage, I would have stayed."

People still speak of us that way.

At first I didn't know how destructive living with chronic illness could be. You can't know until you know. The reality of things creeps up, creeps on, in steps smaller than Ted's. Pretty soon it is two years and then it is ten. Pretty soon you are forty-five and then you are fifty. Ted is still Ted.

We keep changing. Once I was tying Ted's shoes as we got dressed to go to the synagogue for Yom Kippur, the Day of Atonement. He said sharply, "What have I got to atone for?"

Sometimes I forget that deep in his heart he's more religious than I, he sees more of a connection between behavior and reward.

"Nothing." I straightened up. "You don't deserve this rotten disease. You don't deserve it one bit."

"I don't?" He looked relieved.

"No. Not for a minute."

"That's right. I don't."

He seemed to feel better.

So I said it every day for a week.

And I wrote that conversation into the first draft of this book, and added that after a couple of weeks I began to long for Ted to say I didn't deserve MS either, didn't deserve how it had altered my life. But it didn't occur to him.

After he read the draft and finished giving me his comments, he said, "There's one last thing. You don't deserve this rotten disease. You really don't."

Who would leave a man like that?

Ted made it into the 70 percent, into the good statistics. He's still walking. I don't know what lies ahead. In MS, you try not to think ahead. It's too hard, too frightening. I do know I'll never walk down the street with my man, feeling part of an ordinary couple. I'll be holding Ted's hand to support him, or pushing his chair. So we're not an ordinary but an extraordinary couple.

That nice feeling of walking beside a healthy man, I get a few minutes each week when I move along the main street after lunch with various men friends. But Ted is my husband, my binder in time, my home base, the man who knows me best, and I am the woman who knows him best: we are still a pair held together by psychic charges — fewer charges, perhaps, than we would have if he weren't sick, but perhaps no less deep, because sharing the illness becomes itself a charge. We live in the quicksand together. The healthy couple cannot imagine what we know.

# Chapter 18
# Everyday Marriage, Everyday Aging

Some couples manage happy marriages on beyond the traditional two-year glow. Here's how a wife of thirty years puts it:

My husband is a good lover, a good husband, and a good father. I look at a good marriage as a practice of the imagination. Luck counts, the luck of having parents who stayed together well. You've got to believe it's possible. Then you work on it. And you've got to survive the children, the two of you. Don't let them split you up, don't let them get you on opposite sides. After you've survived the children, luck comes in again. I hadn't any idea Frank was so funny when I fell in love with him. I didn't even know I was going to need someone to be funny!

A man married twice explains the difference:

Friendship is the only quality that can keep a marriage worthwhile. If all the other characteristics are present except for friendship, there's no marriage. A lover needs me — or someone like me. But a wife/friend needs me and only me, because for her there *is* no one quite like me.

A woman divorcing describes the pulling apart:

When you're in love you think of the twosome as something benefiting you both. It gives you pleasure to cook for your husband, to set the table, to watch him eat. If the twosome becomes something that destroys you both, you start to hate cooking for him or watching him eat. You hate seeing him walk through the front door. I don't know just how it moves from one stage to another. It may be that supporting children is simply so demanding — or perhaps it's because the two of you have different senses of reality. He may see a child's low mark at school as the fault of the teacher and you may see it as the fault of the child. It's not subject matter. It's an emotional stance. If you fall too far apart in how you each see the world, war sets in.

That's a subjective report. What about an objective report? What makes for happy everyday marriages? We start, in a roundabout way, with family. In the 1960s and 1970s, a long-term study of families at the Timberlawn Psychiatric Research Foundation in Texas revealed no one common denominator in the happy, healthy family, but eight separate variables. Dr. W. Robert Beavers and colleagues published (see Appendix B, under Lewis) the resulting eight-factor scale. The Beavers-Timberlawn scale impressed Florence Kaslow, Ph.D., now a psychologist and family therapist who directs the Florida Couples and Family Institute in West Palm Beach. She adapted (see Appendix B) the family scale for couples and here, paraphrased, are the eight variables that flourishing couples handle well:

1. *They value each other and think of themselves as a unit.* The whole is more than the parts; yet the two aren't symbiotic, neither he nor she is "giving up" anything for the other. The two survive as a twosome in a field of change: periodic negotiations take place. They approve of each other's development and growth. Their harmony is apparent. They give off the sense of valuing each other, they seem to want to please each other. They both believe that if the couple benefits, so does each of them. The unit is open to the world — they behave in a manner that is basically compatible with a larger society and they can seek help or support from outside.

2. *The twosome has boundaries.* The couple is first and last a twosome: they don't need children to define them as parents or parents to define them as children. If their children are grown, they don't long for the old days when the kids were small. They can be apart — both physically and emotionally. They can spend an evening reading or with not-shared friends or take a business trip without accusations. Their sexual needs are met

by each other. Sex means tenderness, passion, and playfulness and is not used as a weapon or to mend conflict.

3. *They talk easily and clearly and act smoothly together.* There are few double-bind messages and few confusions. Neither disparages the other. Both are mentally healthy and able to meet problems creatively. Each allows the other some room in which to disagree, quarrels don't become destructive. Verbal messages match nonverbal messages. Underlying meanings are spoken, not hinted at. There is little stereotyping. They don't mutter; they don't miss each other's words. They hear even fragmented sentences.

4. *They're not engaged in a struggle for power.* There's an equalitarian feel. Neither is taken to be more powerful than the other. The lead shifts, depending on who feels most strongly about a given issue. They don't abdicate power to their children. Each takes responsibility for his or her own thoughts or actions and neither expects the other to read his or her mind. Children sense the strong parental bond and don't separate the parents to make a private bond with one; children don't perceive one good and one bad parent or one right and one wrong: consequently, they don't feel forced into taking sides. Equity, individuality, and happiness are held as higher values than being right or being in charge.

5. *They share a wide range of emotions.* They move from sadness to joy with each other. They feel free to express anger and aren't intimidated by it or by great joy. They have fun together. They share a sense of the absurdity of life. They handle trouble and loss by the free expression of emotions and don't belittle or deny them. They are flexible and innovative and throw out responses that don't work anymore. They try new resources. They don't expect a problem-free life nor do they interpret trouble as a punishment.

6. *They aren't enmeshed, or like Siamese twins.* Each feels whole. Neither is threatened by closeness. They tell each other how they feel, not how the other feels or should feel. Each believes that if the other died, life would still be worth living.

(Elvin Semrad, Boston analyst, professor at Harvard Medical School, and former president of the Boston Psychoanalytic Institute, put it this way [see Appendix B, Rako]: "The more mature a relationship, the more able the two people are to give up their dependency and learn how to live alone together. . . . You can only be close when you're separate.")

7. *They listen to each other and negotiate conflict.* They listen when they hit an impasse, instead of turning out or becoming defensive. They solve problems by hearing everything and trying to work out conflict at the highest level of mutual input. They don't use compromise or conciliation, which so often means someone gives something up.

8. *They share a worldview or value system.* They feel connected to their personal and familial past and future and aren't in conflict with their external environment. They have a belief system that provides meaning and value to life, and connects them with a universal scheme. They are reconciled to mortality, yet they treasure life.

For the well spouse, this reads like a list of the eight areas where we've already experienced trouble. Let's go through it again, adding some of what we know and consulting Dr. Kaslow for her views on how chronic illness changes functioning.

1. *Unit.* The twosome may remain foremost, but its territory shrinks dangerously and the well spouse gives up plenty, as does the sick spouse. Dr. Kaslow emphasizes that with chronic illness "the unit or system has to be very open, particularly to the medical community, perhaps to nursing care. If the couple clings to each other and one spouse says 'I'll do it all,' they deplete themselves."

2. *Boundaries.* Too much enforced closeness threatens the boundaries of individual privacy; sexual needs may not be met; there is great temptation and sometimes the real need to break bonding patterns between parents and children. "It's more tricky to maintain intergenerational boundaries," Dr. Kaslow points out. "And sometimes you can't. If there is too much role reversal, the well spouse becomes more like a parent. It's much more difficult to maintain the privacy dimension if one spouse is dealing with the other's toileting."

"If the sexual function becomes impaired," Dr. Kaslow asks, "how does the healthy partner abstain? That depends on the religious values, on commitment, on how long the period of abstention will be, or age. If the husband or wife is thirty-five and sex is curtailed, my general line of reasoning is to ask one spouse how he or she would want the other to act if the situation were reversed. Sometimes a casual extramarital affair for the well spouse is a way of keeping emotional energy in the marriage. It is important that 'the lover' be told of the marital commitment. I suggest that people act in a way that they can be proud of."

3. *Communication*. This slows if there is deafness or inability to speak, not to mention larger silences. "Sometimes the well spouse should not disclose all," Dr. Kaslow believes, "so as not to destroy the equilibrium of the sick person. But it's good to have as much open communication as you can handle: otherwise the illness controls the couple."

4. *Equality*. Although there may be no intentional struggle for power, the basic equality shifts as the sick person becomes far more dependent on the well. "It's so difficult to maintain equality," Dr. Kaslow confirms, "where one is taking care of the other. If the patient takes the best possible care of himself, that's good. If he or she doesn't try to manage the illness, there will be a far greater disturbance of the egalitarian relationship and two things can happen. The well partner may take too much control or the sick spouse may use the illness to control the well. The patient may say 'how can you go out and leave me alone?' The well partner becomes the captive. This gives the patient tremendous power."

5. *Emotional range*. The desired wide range of emotion may shrink as fears and sorrows, angers and guilts, are denied and as joy, hope, and pleasure abate. The sick person may become falsely cheerful and the well one may bear the couple's depression. Constantly coping beyond capacity, the well person may withdraw from emotional expression, too. "A full range of emotion should continue," Dr. Kaslow urges. "It's important that the couple be sad and grieve and share pleasures."

6. *Autonomy*. This may collapse. For example, the stroke victim loses one kind of autonomy, the Alzheimer's victim another. In attempting to compenstate, the well partner invades the sick's internal space and the sick intrudes upon the well for help. "The sick person should keep as much autonomy as possible," Dr. Kaslow says without hesitation: "writing the letters, doing the checks, keeping records, making phone calls — whatever that partner can still do. The sick partner should not make the healthy partner's life more involved with the illness than necessary."

7. *Negotiation*. This may hold — if it was there to start. Perhaps, however, a couple was still growing in this and other areas. The added demands of chronic illness may halt a

couple's growth. "A couple should keep task negotiation as close to normal as possible. The sick partner needs not to be indulged or pampered, but encouraged to function at the highest possible level."

8. *Shared values.* The shared value system sounds good, but when one is dying considerably faster than the other, reconciliation to mortality comes down to the difference between "I'm dying" and "You're dying." Perceptions about mortality split. "A shared transcendental value system can carry people through much adversity," Dr. Kaslow maintains, "no matter which value system it is. This can really help."

You do the best you can. Illness really does skew a marrige, yet some of your troubles may lie in the twosome that preexisted the illness. Happy marriages imply a union of two happy, well-adjusted people. You may each have to grow individually. Take a closer look at those eight variables. Figure out where you're weakest and how to change. If you're scoring a pitiful 4 on the 8 points, take heart. So, probably, are most everyday couples.

How do couples with a chronic illness manage the twosome? Empathy helps. Earlier, in chapter 6, we tried to avoid looking at the world through the sick person's eyes. But that was only to keep a grip on ourselves, only to establish that we, too, exist. For actually living with someone, empathy remains key. Miriam uses lots of it; she's also very positive and practices a real thanksgiving. "I made a rule," she explained in her opening remarks, "that we couldn't talk about Daniel's pain while we were eating, particularly during dessert." Before you start feeling guilty that you're not so positive as Miriam, consider this: Daniel's mobile; they've a good sexual life; he supports them, even though he lost his job and now works from home. Are they happy because they had a good marriage to start? Or because Daniel's illness is less catastrophic than others?

> Even with a good relationship (which is what we have), the constant, daily encounter can be wearing. We snap at each other much more than we ever did. It isn't like me, and it isn't like Daniel. I wonder sometimes what has happened to my patience; sometimes I feel as if I've shorted out. I get cross and irritable. Little things drive me wild. Emptying matches from the ashtrays (Daniel smokes a pipe) or changing the toilet paper roll (it's hard

for Daniel to bend over and do it). And yet when he says, "I'll get the mail today," I get annoyed because I know how much it takes out of him and it seems like a waste of his good energy. I'd rather sit on the sofa and talk with him about the future of social studies, the Regents Action Plan, or tutoring young Ralph, a challenging job that we have both taken on together.

It could be worse, that big, gaping hole that is the worst — without Daniel, the Daniel I love and cannot live without. I don't see it as weakness, I recognize the inextricableness, doubleness, intertwined nature of our relationship. This morning I woke up at 6:00. Daniel was sleeping. His labored breathing troubles me, and that cough, deep, persistent, his lungs trying hard for more breathing space as the postpolio finds its way around his body. I try to take these signs in stride, not to be afraid. I take pleasure in the gift of moments. Such a handsome man. I'm filled with pleasure at the sight of him. I stroke his face, he murmers from somewhere deep in his unconscious. Out the window, the willow trees are radiant with spring, a gentle yellow powdering through the network of brown branches. This is a blessing. I take it hungrily, this moment — with its peace, and wonder, and its quiet joy.

Steve's account reads with that same sense of pleasure in and respect for the person he married. He and Jerilyn married at twenty and nineteen, when Steve had little idea of how serious Type I diabetes can be. Jerilyn handled her illness very well, very strictly. They lost their first child hours after she was born. They had two more children and, much later, a third. When they were thirty-seven and thirty-six, Jerilyn began to lose her sight. This strained the equality of the twosome, and although they both got angrier than in the past, the anger didn't turn into domestic war.

During one period Steve took time out from his job as an accountant to travel from Maine to Boston for Jerilyn's laser treatments. She endured three sight-restoring operations with nothing but Novocaine, but each time she eventually lost her sight again. At forty, she was completely blind. Steve speaks:

I said to myself, It's not fair. I've had my share, I don't want any more. Yet when she started losing her sight, I was very supportive, I felt closer to her — I don't know why. I had to be there to give her all my strength and words of encouragement.

I wasn't really thinking of myself then, I hadn't realized this was here to stay.

She would go into her room and feel depressed, which I could understand. But she'd be in there without lights. She didn't want to talk to me and that really upset me. She needed this time for herself, but it went on too long. I felt she had to accept the blindness. Until she accepted it, I couldn't accept it. I yelled at her to get out of the rut, to go on with our lives.

The Blind Association made weekly visits and she learned to walk with a white cane. She wanted to be independent. She was very stubborn. The Association was terrific; they brought her stickers for her washer and dryer, they taught her how to do all her housework without sight.

We fought more. She was so meticulous and it meant a lot to her. I didn't know what to do sometimes. I'd go behind her at supper and pick up what she missed. Carrot peelings in the sink, for instance. How could she see those? But I had to sneak them out because she got mad if she knew I was going behind her.

She couldn't measure her insulin and I had to do it and it made me nervous so I did it slow and that made her upset. So we'd have an argument.

Grocery shopping was a real challenge. We'd walk in and by the second or third aisle we'd be fighting.

"Do you need stewed tomatoes?" I'd say.

"Well . . ." She'd take a long time to think about it. She couldn't visualize what was on the shelves anymore.

I missed my work out in the yard. But I stayed inside and vacuumed the floor and picked up the kids' stuff so she wouldn't fall over it. The doctors restricted sexual activities after one operation, but we've got a lot of love for one another and once things could resume to normal, there was no problem, none at all.

When Jerilyn was first blind she didn't want to go out. I wanted her to and I wanted her to look good. I was always concerned she didn't look blind, I always wanted her to look like she was Jerilyn. I would tell her, "You need some lipstick and a little makeup." I helped her put it on, the eyeshadow, too, and we would go to dinner or dancing, and the more she did, the easier it got. I figured this was the way it was going to be and I accepted it.

And it was that way for three years. Then she had a fourth

operation and, so far, she can see. The arguments are fewer. I tend to my yard. She drives by day and I by night. Lately I've begun to take it for granted. Perhaps too much so, but I would hate to think we'd have to got back to that way of living again.

I'd do it over. We've had a good married life. The only thing is that when I hear people complaining about some tiny problem I think, 'Boy, you don't have a problem!' To sum it up, if you love one another as much as we do and you've vowed to honor and obey in sickness and in health, it's all there. I know if I had the problem, she would treat me with every loving care she could possibly give me.

In upstate New York, Laurie is only four years older than Steve, but her life stage measures out differently. At fifty-one, Laurie has launched two children into marriage with her husband, Bill, who is sixty-two. She's nearing the end of thirty years of a happy marriage.

I'm married to the most wonderful husband anybody ever had, and I am watching him die slowly and unpleasantly.

He waited five years for me to grow up (to twenty-one) and marry him. He was honest with me; he told me he'd been in a sanatorium for lung disease and that it had been arrested. We were so much in love. It never occurred to us that smoking was the last thing he should have been doing.

Gradually over the years I learned about his physical limitations, but more important, I learned how much he loved me. Enough never to criticize me, never to correct me, never to laugh at my mistakes — enough to accept me totally, exactly the way I was, with all of my faults. Slowly by example he taught me how to be a mature human being.

In 1983, when he was diagnosed as having chronic obstructive pulmonary disease, I got most of the crying out of my system while the staff was trying to save him. I asked God to let him have a little more time and God very kindly responded; I was terrified when I brought him home. I was sure that I would soon be a widow.

Gradually his Irish stubbornness asserted itself, and two months after he came home we decided that a new motorcycle would be a real incentive. His Suzuki looked a little odd with the portable oxygen tank strapped on the rear carrier, but we managed. Motorcycle riding, curiously enough, doesn't require a lot of physical effort, and the rider assumes a position which is quite comfortable for someone with breathing problems.

Because my husband's activities had always been somewhat limited, my adjustment to his illness wasn't made as abruptly as other people's. The most difficult part was coming to grips with what I perceived as the primary cause of his illness — his addiction to cigarettes. I would not allow myself to say to him, "I told you so." What good would it do? At first this did nothing to stop my anger toward his one weakness. Although I had once threatened several years ago, when I began to detect signs of respiratory disease, to leave him if he didn't give up the habit, I could not now leave him and would not if I had the chance. I know that if our roles were reversed, he would unquestioningly take care of me. I could not do less for him.

It's strange how some positive things have come out of this. I've found that I'm a lot tougher than I ever thought I was; I found confidence in abilities that I might never have discovered if I hadn't been forced into it. I've learned to plant a garden. I've become more assertive with the bureaucratic obstacles that stand between my husband and his comfort. I thought I knew what love was when we married. The Reverend Billy Graham has recently described genuine love as an "act of the will." I'm beginning to know what he means.

You do some serious thinking, have some serious dialogue, and ask whoever is in charge of throwing fast curves, How can I do better by this man? Maybe it's prayer, but not the kind you find in the back of the hymnal. You have to consciously remind yourself of how you would react or how you would feel in his situation. Bill makes me feel like Wonder Woman and Raquel Welch rolled into one. When this is all over, I am going to have a lot of time to remember. And I don't want to remember any more bad things than I have to. I don't want the last part of our marriage to overshadow the earlier part. His time should be as happy as I can make it. I only hope I have the strength and the guts to keep on trying.

If your marriage pales beside these, it may be that the twosome had troubles to start. Or it may be that the illness you're dealing with demands more. What would happen if Daniel could no longer work? If Jerilyn went blind again? If Laurie were a trial lawyer who needed to travel? If Bill had a thirty-year life expectancy? If Daniel and Miriam had children and their budget required full-time work from Miriam? If any of the sick spouses were losing their wits? But trouble isn't the focus in this chapter. What we want to witness here is the relative ease with which these happily married couples throw off the angrier and more divisive emotions of chronic illness and with what agility they keep clear of total collapse. In this respect they are blessed.

— ◆ —

## A CHECKLIST FOR THE SICK SPOUSE

(Remember: You don't deserve to be sick.)

1. Do you feel guilty? Inadequate? Deprived? Scared? Angry? When was the last time you spoke these feelings to your spouse? To someone else? To yourself? In other words, have you truly mourned your loss? If you keep stoically quiet, your spouse may feel that he or she can't have bad feelings about it either. Being too stoical sets it up so that others around you must be equally stoical or else express all the bad emotions while you do only the cheer.

2. Do you rely on your spouse to be your only friend? When was the last time you called a friend of your own? Made a new friend?

3. Do you ask your spouse for help without noticing what he or she is already doing? Is your spouse on the way to that very task? In the middle of another? True, you feel frustrated, but imagine what it's like to be somebody else's arms and legs.

4. Do you take your spouse for granted? Or distrust your spouse? Worry that you'll be abandoned? Neither extreme feels good to the other person.

5. Have you urged your spouse to do alone some of the things you can no longer do together — such as going to the movies, skiing, swimming?

6. Did you notice how your spouse was feeling at suppertime? Not in regard to you, just in general? For an acute sickness, it's natural to be self-occupied and oblivi-

ous to the feelings of others. If you're chronically self-occupied, it's pretty tough on the rest of us.

7. Do you trust your spouse to act with both your best interests at heart? And in doing so, to sometimes choose his or her own needs over yours?

8. Do you ever leave the nasty little things, such as calling Blue Cross, to your spouse on the grounds that you're sick?

9. When was the last time you yourself planned something fun for the two of you to do together? If this week, you have won the heart of every reader.

10. When was the last time you talked with your spouse about how she or he would manage financially if you died? If you had to live in a nursing home?

11. When was the last time your spouse told you his or her real fears?

12. Have you called your spouse a workaholic lately? Unduly pessimistic? Bossy and controlling? That could be your guilt speaking. Do you take as much responsibility as possible?

13. Did you do something charming today?

14. Think of three wonderful moments in your life together.

---

## A CHECKLIST FOR THE WELL SPOUSE

(Remember: It really is worse to be sick.)

1. Have you truly mourned the old marriage and made up your mind about the viability of the new? What's in it for you? Have you made as much of a life for yourself as you want? If you haven't, how much can you fairly blame on the illness?

2. How's your empathy? Do you really know your spouse's physical limitations? Which of them bothered him or her most today? Do you really know the level of your spouse's sense of guilt? Fear? Dependence? Have

you tried to find out (books, doctor, support groups) the emotions that the disease commonly brings out?

3. What are the things you hate about your spouse? Which of them are due to the illness? Which are not? Don't overlook the effect of drugs or of speeded-up aging or of economic decline.

4. Did you find time today to really connect with him or her? Pressures aside, anger aside, did you manage to drop all that and connect for just a few seconds, in a laugh, for instance? Take 100 points!

5. Did you make a unilateral decision today that you suspect he or she would really have liked a share in? Are you doing more than you really have to? Infantilizing him or her?

6. In which ways do you still feel like a member of an equal twosome?

7. Do you speak clearly? Or do you expect your spouse to read your mind? Are you afraid to say what you mean? Do your words match your body language? Do you manage to avoid telling your spouse what he or she feels? (Good!) Do you dare to get mad at him or at her? At someone *sick?* Do you acquiesce or compromise more than you want to? Where do the two of you fall off the Beavers-Timberlawn scale? How could you yourself change?

8. Where have you polarized? Do you, for instance, overstate the negative and your spouse the positive? Maybe it's because your spouse denies or ignores reality, but try for balance in your own statements and see what happens.

9. Have you asked your spouse for help today?

10. Do you believe your spouse could get well if he or she changed attitudes or diet? Is your belief realistic?

11. Are you more fused as a couple than you would like? What have you done for fun by yourself this week?

12. Do you respect your spouse? If not, how could you get your respect back?

13. Remember three happy moments you've had to-gether.

———◄◉►———

# Chapter 19
# What Lies Ahead?

"We'll get divorced if I have to go into a nursing home," Ted said one autumn Sunday after Seth had gone to college, as he sat at the dining table reading the Sunday *Times*.

"What?" I was in the kitchen sprinkling wheat germ on the apple crisp.

"There's a piece in the *Times* — you can't go into a nursing home if you've got more than some tiny sum in the bank."

I opened the oven door. "No. We won't get divorced."

Why should the words sting so?

They just did. They sounded sad. Sad words.

"You'd visit me every day." He looked up as I walked into the dining room. "I'd still love you."

I put my arms around him. "I'd still love you." I sat at the round table where I'd eaten alone years ago in the city, wondering why I wasn't married.

"You'll never have to go to a nursing home." I picked up the article. But what if I couldn't afford nurses? There will never be enough money for me to retire. I'll be working until I fall. What if I had to work and nurse Ted, too? I'd promised Jane I wouldn't. It might come to that, a nursing home. After all, we had Medicare.

The article said Medicare doesn't cover nursing homes. Only Medicaid does, and if you have to put your spouse in, you lose everything you've saved, maybe even the house. I couldn't swallow. This meant there would be no end. No matter what I did, the sickness would never end. Even if Ted died, I would be paying my dues to MS because I'd have spent all my resources and become totally dependent.

"That's what I meant." Ted folded the page for our file.

"He'll never have to go to a nursing home," Susan assured me in her small Boston kitchen before the Thanksgiving meal. We'll all pool what we have. We'll all take care of him together."

Could I nurse Ted at sixty and sixty-five and seventy? Would Susan be there for breakfast, lunch, and dinner? Would the kids spend their holidays nursing Dad?

"Seth looks wonderful!" Susan said.

And he did, a young man, assured. "This month I walked down to the Battery," he told the dozen at the table around the turkey. "At first I walked around the Upper West Side where we used to live. But now I walk all over the city."

Across the table from me Debbie listened to Seth. "I haven't talked much about Dad's being sick," she'd finally confided in me on our trip to an art school in Pennsylvania, "because it's somehow hard and humiliating to admit you're scared. The worst thing is that I don't know Dad so well now. I haven't had enough serious talks with him. I can't separate the illness from the real personality. Sometimes we still have fun, sometimes at the dinner table. But it's rare. One of us is usually mad at something. The anger comes from the sickness. Dad gets angry because he's sick. You get angry because you have the most work to do. We're still kids and we don't want to deal with this while we're growing up. Neither should either of you have to deal with it, but the fact is, we do have to. It's changed all our personalities. I guess the worst part is feeling alienated or estranged from Dad."

Maybe someday this would change; but that wouldn't erase what had happened. As Debbie put it, "You can't change the past."

"I got all the way to Fourteenth Street and it started to rain." Seth continued to the table. He did not possess a coat, refused to possess one. Probably the result of our forcing him into snowsuits when he was little. You do what you can. He, too, had broken his silence one noontime in a Chinese restaurant. "If Dad weren't sick the whole family would be less tense. He's tense all the time and we're tense all the time." Our life, he said, had resembled that in the movie *Fun with Dick and Jane*. "They were just putting in the swimming pool when Dick gets fired and they have to turn to crime to keep things up. But it wasn't the money that mattered. It was the drop in interesting things. We stopped doing things, we stopped seeing people. This wasn't all because of the illness. Aunt Susan got divorced. Uncle Bob got divorced. We'd moved. Mostly I get annoyed, but I don't feel guilty anymore. You cheapened guilt — making me mow the lawn when you wanted. A lawn should run a little wild. The main thing is the general paternal collapse followed by the responsibilities shifting. Three people are taking care of a fourth. The three are cranky about that and the fourth is cranky about being sick."

How would they feel at thirty or fifty?

"Next week, I'm trying the Lower East Side." Seth wound up his description.

Ted's eyes met mine: he used to walk all over the city, too, when he was young.

The children mustn't be responsible for us.

Or for me.

Debbie stopped seeing Dr. Rose after a few sessions in the spring of her sophomore year. When her first junior marks came in shortly after Thanksgiving, she started seeing a math tutor and an English tutor, Thea. It was my friend Thea who figured it out.

"I've noticed that when she talks or listens, she gets every nuance," Thea explained as we sat with our feet over the edge of the YMCA pool. "She's very bright. But when it comes to reading something complex in small print, she balks. Is she comfortable, do you think, when she reads? I was wondering about her eyes?"

Her eyes!

"Her English teacher wonders, too," Thea continued. "He says she tries, but if she can't do the first part of something, she chucks the whole thing."

I swam back and forth, back and forth, and when I got to my office, I dialed up a friend in New York who works with dyslexia and other vision-related problems. "Parts and wholes, trouble with managing time, reading small dense print . . ."

"Yes," the friend said. "Go to the library. Read."

I found several case studies of cross-eyed children showing academic histories like Debbie's, but her surgeon in New York told me this was poppycock. Still, I made a date for consultation with a New York optometrist and vision trainer. Meanwhile, our local ophthalmologist filled Debbie's earlier prescription from her New York surgeon for contact lenses. The lenses hadn't anything to do with near-point vision, but they would equalize her near and far eye for distance. To my surprise, this doctor remarked that Debbie suffered from severe eyestrain: "Life will be easier for her now," he said, in his doorway.

She started wearing her contacts that February, the weekend I drove her to the Cape to look for summer jobs. She took the wheel out of Hyannis and drove for ten minutes in her black Eurofashion with her hair slicked back and her sunglasses covering the lenses — radio blaring.

"Wow! This is terrific!" she called over the noise. "I don't have a piercing headache. Without my lenses, I'd feel all tense by now because I'd have a terrible headache!" She drove one hundred miles and never got the headache.

Why hadn't I known? The surgeon's obfuscation? My constant distraction and overwork? The school's preconceptions blocking any other investigation? Everybody's blaming the MS? If there had been no illness at home, wouldn't we all have investigated more broadly sooner? We must make more room in our lives for the rest of the family. It can't be just Ted.

I, too, needed to be able to look ahead without getting a headache. A support group for the spouses of people with MS finally opened an hour's drive from us. Four women sat in the room when I entered. Two were younger than I and two older. One of the older women was talking, Marianne: "I met a woman at a doctor's office once who told me I'd get to the point when if he fell, I'd step right over him and move on. I was so shocked. But I am here tonight to tell you that I've reached that point. I've stepped right over him."

The younger woman and I exchanged looks. Oooh, this was stiff. We didn't ever want to be this angry at our husbands!

White-haired Eleanor had a soft voice and tears came easily to her eyes. "When I visit him in the nursing home, he has nothing for me, nothing. He never even asks how I am. I don't feel married at all. It takes me an hour to get there and I go every afternoon to feed him supper. When he does talk, he only complains about the nurses. He can flick the TV button, that's all. For me it's all give, give, give, and for him it's all take, take, take. I know I should do more for myself. But I feel so guilty. . . ." Her eyes filled with tears.

The two younger women and I exchanged looks again. Oooh, this wasn't right, either. We didn't want to become total martyrs to our husbands.

We all avoided each other as we walked to the parking lot.

At the second meeting, Eleanor told how her greatest help had been a parish priest. Now that he had died, she was lonelier than ever, but her religion kept her afloat. Once in her kitchen when she was still nursing her husband at home she had seen Jesus holding a basin of water. This wordless picture reminded her and repersuaded her that the humblest acts — even the washing of somebody's feet — can be holy. She didn't cry when she told this story: the image gave her strength. She also reported that she'd joined a volunteer group to read to the blind.

Marianne described how her husband had changed in the eighteen years of his MS. It had all come together for her one night five years ago when she'd caught the flu. With fever and chills, she decided to sleep in another room so her husband wouldn't catch the flu. He wouldn't let her. He told her to get herself a face mask and sleep on a mattress on the floor by his bed. She mustn't leave him. Lying down there on the mattress, she realized that her husband was no longer the gentle, considerate man she'd married: there'd been personality changes.

After that meeting we all walked to Marianne's car to see the sling and hoist by which she gets her husband in and out.

At the third meeting, Eleanor said she'd gone to the movies with a friend.

Marianne described her day. It begins when she, like Kathy in Georgia, gets her husband via a mechanical lift from his bed into his TV chair. Then she drives to the computer store where she works. At lunch she goes home to feed her husband and catheterize him and get him back into bed via the lift. The clerks at the store can always tell if she's had a bad time at noon. They're terrific. They bolster her up. Her kids come to visit a bit, but she long ago vowed that the illness wouldn't change their lives more than necessary. Even so, her daughter stayed at home a long time helping out before she married. Her son is an angrier young man than Marianne wishes: "All his emotion turned into anger." He left early and married young. Now he comes by to mow the lawn, apologizing for his adolescent refusals to do so. At the store, Marianne watches the clock until five.

Some days she has to talk herself home. "Come on now," she says to herself from the office door all the way to the parking lot. "Come on now, you can do it," all the way home. Her husband's friends stopped coming as he stopped making contact. He can't talk. When she comes in, he glances at his watch. "This is supposed to mean he's pissed at me. I'm five minutes late. Then he hits the wall by the bed with his cane. It's the only movement he can make, a small lateral movement. There's a big hole in the plaster from where he hits it."

The two younger women and I looked at each other: so there is no escape. We are one with Marianne; we are one with Eleanor. Their two extremes are just the two extremes of the end game. Their husbands' MS had simply progressed further than our husbands'. Given their conditions, we'd probably grow even angrier or even more self-denying. Eleanor was doing pretty darn well. Marianne, too. As it turned out, Marianne wasn't even older than I but exactly my age: she just looked older. This was the future.

After the third meeting, we all embraced in the lobby.

We "younger" three had been strangers lost in Asia. Crossing the steppes, we'd stumbled upon two English-speaking travelers and been relieved to hear that they knew the same nouns as we did, the same verbs. We spoke the same language and didn't have to apologize for or explain our pronunciation. We could ask Marianne and Eleanor for directions.

But could we bear to hear them?


When I got home, Ted and Nick with his new woman friend, Claire, and Nellie were in the dining room playing Hearts. Nick cut me some of the bread he'd brought and Nellie ladled out her soup.

I dealt the next hand.

After a few games, Nick put down our scores: a winning 40 for himself, 50 for me, 62 for Nellie, 65 for Claire, and a trailing 81 for Ted.

"You wouldn't treat a poor cripple like that," Ted whined in an artificial voice. "A handicapped person should have a handicap."

"Bug off!" we all shouted, in one whoop.

A nice balance, on this rung.

Later in the winter, Ted lay in bed and said, "I don't want to go on living past the point where I'm in too bad shape."

"Are you talking about suicide?" I turned toward him.

"Yes."

"Don't. Please don't. Please don't ever talk about it." Two of my cousins had done it. It's too awful, too creepy. I'd decided against it years ago, no matter what. The children of suicides are more prone. I'd never do it.

"I have to think about it."

"Well, I can't think about it, ever!"

Debbie spent a week with a friend while we visited Doris on a senior preserve in Florida. To escape the strip and mall landscape, we drove one afternoon to a corner of the Everglades. We boarded an airboat, choosing the small shade offered by the boat's propelling device — a gigantic rotary fan that screeched and vibrated while warming up. The tour guide passed out cotton batten for our ears, but Ted eschewed his.

With terrific noise, the boat took off. The guide began his spiel about the words "Ever — Glades" scrawled on an early explorer's map of the area. We moved over the face of the waters, scaring off long-legged birds that rose nonetheless gracefully at our ominous approach. The guide killed the fan when he spotted a touristy-looking alligator sunning itself motionless on a tiny sharp-edged island. In half an hour we finished our tour and settled back at the dock.

"I can't hear anything." Ted spoke hollowly as the guide and I helped him out of the boat.

"It'll wear off," the guide assured him.

We sat on Doris's balcony overlooking golf carts and a tropical sunset.

"What did you say?" Ted looked up from the real estate ads he loves to examine in other city's papers.

"Supper's ready," I shouted.

The next night we watched a televised *Rigoletto* as we sat on Doris's enormous, although now single, bed. "What were those words?"

*"Weep, weep my child, let your tears fall upon my heart."* I repeated them and shut off the air conditioning in case that

might help. Ted's hearing wasn't improving at all. Was he going to lose hearing next? Stunning, a stunning loss.

Would I now become his senses, not just his hands and legs and fingers? Stunning, a stunning possibility.

"Turn it up again, will you?" Ted's pale legs lay on the bed, his right foot red and swollen.

I couldn't believe it. My sorrow for Ted's hearing faded into a growing panic and rage. He was climbing right into my body. I was climbing right into his, into his sensory lobes, into his auditory cortex and he into mine. This was a gradual total body transplant in which my own self would be entirely usurped.

Doris asked me what was the matter and walked me gently around the condo's entrance paths while I tried to control the tears of hopelessness that ran out of my eyes.

"There were things . . ." — I searched for ways to put it — "that I once wanted . . . to do . . ." I stopped. This was Doris's son.

A week after we got home Ted could hear again.

Debbie dyed the tips of her short glossy hair a straw yellow. Seth returned at spring break, taller, freer, a semifinished product.

"Do you think you'll major in medieval studies?" Ted inquired as we sat around the table with the rosy curtains drawn.

"Mayhap." Seth didn't give it away, using Ted's old deadpan approach.

"You do seem suited to it." Ted didn't crack a smile either, although there was a distinct brightening of his eyes.

The old guerrilla warfare, as the poet Linda Pastan calls it, seemed ended.

"I don't ever want to be a vegetable." Ted brought it up again. He lay on the cot on the porch as the dogwood blossomed. "What if I couldn't move? Or talk? Or hear? What if I couldn't scratch my nose? I'd tell you with one flick of an eyelid to scratch my nose. With two, to call the doctor. And we could have a special signal. Three flicks means it's time to do me in."

"Sure. I always wanted to spend the golden years in jail." The white blossoms of the tree shone like Easter lilies. The buzz of spring whispered all its promises.

"That's why I have to do it before I'm paralyzed."

"Forget it, I'm not murdering you."

In Boston's Kenmore Square, a pair of optometrists found Debbie's first two surgeries so clean and free of scars that they would accept her for binocular vision training. The New York specialist who had referred us to Boston said Debbie should get her written information through the ear, by tape, until she learned to fuse. What changes might fusion bring?

"You probably noticed," the younger Boston doctor said, "that when she came in she sat down in the chair with her toes pointing in, her knees together and in, her head down, and her shoulders hunched, like this." He sat and gave a perfect picture of the posture that had for years caused professionals and friends to point out that Debbie was very, very depressed. "That's how strabismics sit. The wall-eyed sit like this." He demonstrated the opposite posture. "It's just our observation. We haven't got statistics to prove it, but we have also noticed that if we straighten out the eyes, the posture tends to straighten."

They hovered over Debbie, measured angles, listed numbers, showed excitement about their work — her first positive feedback for her troubled eyes. Whether their program accomplished all the goals we wished or not, it ought to be good for her. Outside, Debbie and I walked to the square where she was meeting a friend from an art school. I asked how she liked the doctors.

"It's a new field," she explained in her wonderful combination of adolescent and wise woman. "They have to learn from the patients. We're all they've got. I'll do it."

When her black-clothed friend arrived, I went into a bookstore.

Asking for Derek Humphry's *Jean's Way* at your local store feels like buying your first sanitary napkins from six boys in your homeroom with after-school jobs. I found the book and stood, skimming. After a mastectomy and radiation, Humphry's wife's cancer spread to the bones. She told him she wanted to die by her own choice when she was ready. She asked him to find the means. How could he deny her? He found the right mixture of Seconal and codeine from a doctor friend. The day came. He brought the cup on a tray. After fifty minutes, she died in her sleep. He called the doctor and went for a walk in the garden. When he published his account of this, Britain's Director of Public Prosecution ordered an investigation, but a groundswell of public opinion . . . I put the book back. I picked up Humphry's next book, *Let Me Die Before I Wake*, and paid for it.

I sat at Dunkin' Donuts in the spring rain and read. One suffering man's wife was too frightened of widowhood to let him kill himself: me. Too clingy, she even threatened to do herself in if he killed himself: selfish me. His death was painful and prolonged. At Dunkin' Donuts, I changed my mind. I took out my pencil and circled all the footnoted dosages that the people Humphry interviewed had tried. That way I would never again have to pass my eyes over such accounts as that of a daughter obeying her mother's request and smothering her with a plastic bag — watching her mother's contorting face go purple under the plastic.

Reading a book like Humphry's quite changes the world. The decision was Ted's, but I would no longer stand in Ted's way. I hid the book under the tires in the trunk, and as we drove west in the darkness I began to tell Debbie the history of the world as I knew it. I finished Paleolithic and stopped for a breath.

"Why," she asked me, "if the moon is shining in the light of the sun — which we can't see now because it's on the other side of us — why are the edges of the moon so sharp?"

Clearly, I'd never had all the answers.

"Write away and get me one of those living wills, the kind you got my parents, will you?" Ted sat at the wrought iron table on the porch, after the lilacs faded and the dogwood bloomed.

"I could Xerox a living will for you out of this nifty little book I bought. I tells how to do yourself in." I waited. Maybe he really wanted me to object. If so, I'd never mention the book again.

"What book?" His face filled with a look of exquisite consciousness. "Tell me."

So I told him about Humphry, about the book, and about the Hemlock Society in Los Angeles.

"Good." He kept that same look, relaxing. "Bring it out before you go, okay?" I was leaving soon for New York to fetch Seth and his stereo home for the summer.

"Don't read it alone," I warned him as I set the black book with the yellow butterfly on the porch table.

"You did." He looked up at me, the eyes light in his wry, ironic face.

So we became grown-ups together.

Equals, again.

Chapter 20

# Till Death
## Does or Doesn't
## Us Part

How will it end? Will he be paralyzed? Will she forget her own name? Will you be feeding and cleaning your spouse? Some 13 percent of home nursing for the older frail (see Appendix B, Stone) is provided by husbands, but more often it's wives who nurse.

In 1980 the newly founded Older Women's League commissioned a report on home nursing. It emerged as *Till Death Do Us Part: Caregiving Wives of Severely Disabled Husbands* (see Appendix B, Colman). "It is the wives, who are usually younger than the men they marry, who are carrying the tremendous burden of caring for their older husbands . . ." the report runs. "The caregiving wife . . . is asked to take on an overwhelming task without public support. She is saving taxpayer money, but her own concerns are not taken into account. She is the invisible victim of an inequitable and thoroughly inadequate system. . . . Women interviewed often state that while a doctor will help a man find assistance in caring for an invalid, brain-damaged wife, he will send a husband in the same condition home to his wife with such words as, 'Isn't he lucky to have a wonderful woman like you to take care of him!' "

Vanda Colman found the subjects for this report in two San Francisco area support groups. Women Who Care, in Marin County, was founded by a wife who had taken care of her husband — a stroke victim — for fifteen years. The Family Survival Project in San Francisco gives support and information to the families of people with brain damage.

"There was one man whose wife had Alzheimer's," Colman recalls, as she sits in her living room in front of a window overlooking the white houses of San Francisco and the great blue bay. "He was still working and couldn't afford to hire help. So he rigged up his garage to make what was basically a padded cell where she'd be safe. He put her in there every morning and took her out every evening. He did the best he could.

"All my subjects coped. They varied in denial and in the kinds of illnesses they were dealing with, but they all coped. Their knee joints were disintegrating, their discs were acting up, and their blood pressure rising, but they went on. When one woman finally gave in and put her husband into a nursing home, she noticed how many men were there. Their wives had died.

"It's six years now but I remember the poignancy of those women, the pity of their isolation, the children who had disappeared. Especially sons." Colman adds, "Daughters didn't really stick, either. Also, friends melt away. Particularly when it's Alzheimer's. People with strokes just sit. But people with Alzheimer's get violent. Their brains may be gone, but their bodies are strong and mobile, very mobile.

"A tiny, bright-eyed woman who'd been very close with her husband told me that he would pick up furniture to heave at her. She'd distract him. 'Oh, look!' she'd say, pointing behind him. He had such a short attention span that he would drop the chair and look around. It was awful for her to watch the disintegration of the man she loved.

"Another woman," Colman continues, "had developed heart disease and a bad back from lifting her husband, who had survived a stroke. She needed surgery herself. She hefted him in and out of his wheelchair, fed him, dressed him, shaved him. She got out only once a week and that was to come to the support group meeting. There she found a bit of social life and even a friend who once helped her deal with her husband's blocked bowels. Together they handled what turned out to be an eight-hour enema.

"These women were each other's mainstay. The only human

voice some of them heard in a week was when they went to the grocery store and the clerk said, 'How are you?' Yet they gave a marvelous Christmas party for each other.

"They were loyal. They didn't want to put their husbands into nursing homes. What they needed was respite care. Someone to come in for a week. Or someplace to which they could transport their husbands for a break. The way it is now, these women don't live. The ones I saw pretty much just existed. They really had no energy for anything else but the support group. It's a fate worse than death for these women," Colman concludes. "They shouldn't have to work that hard. They shouldn't have to worry, 'How will I live after he dies?' Or 'Will they take my house if I put him in a nursing home?' It's not right. It's just not right."

Why is home nursing in vogue? "There's been a longstanding romance about very sick people dying at home," reflects Margaret Gold, Ph.D., a sociologist affiliated with the Mount Sinai School of Medicine and with the Brookdale Center on Aging in New York. "The image of the patient lying back on soft pillows, surrounded by loving friends, family, and maybe a favorite pet on the afghan — who wouldn't want to end their days that way? Policymakers didn't pay much attention to the romance of home care until the last decade and the desperate need to cut hospital costs. Home care began to look like a pretty good idea. The ideology of the 'good death at home' got pressed into the service of economy. The catch is — if enough of the right kind of assistance doesn't follow the patient home from the hospital, the romance can turn into a nightmare. Home care is a terrible strain on spouses and families. Yet what you hear from some government agencies these days is concern about sending too much help into the home because it might 'undermine the family's caregiving capacity'!"

Demoralizing as it may be to look ahead to the later stages of your spouse's illness, a long look now is vital. As you read the following letters from a fifty-nine-year-old woman in Indianapolis, ask yourself whether you would be able to live this life. Liz married Carlo knowing his stiff gait and slightly slurred speech came from a bout of multiple sclerosis suffered as a teenager. She loved him and they were both fond of hard work, reading, the arts, and music. They raised two children while Carlo's illness progressed very, very slowly. Then, in his fifties, he broke an arm and a hip and everything went downhill from there on.

*July 17, 1985.* I am just sitting down and *making* the time to write to you as I've been thinking of doing so for eons. It is six years since Carlo's fall, and he is now sitting in his bed watching TV.

I'll give you a typical rundown. We get up anywhere between 6 and 8 A.M. I get his leg bag and take off his night bag, and clean it in the basement. Then we struggle to get him on the walker. Sometimes he falls and I have to help lift him. He has about fifty lbs. on me so it is a chore! Slowly we *inch* to the bathroom. He is taking so few and such small steps that we often have him sit along the route. We generally get him to the bath seat whilst he hangs on the grab bar. We remove his undershirt and jocks as he couldn't sleep in pajamas. Then he must sit until I can help him onto the bath seat in the tub. We wash. Then we get him out, and dried. He dresses himself partially (in a robe, street clothes are too hard) and I help with any difficult parts. He must sit and rest. Then the "fun" begins. Slowly, we inch with the walker to the kitchen. When he gets to the chair we are lucky if he sits on it and not beside it. It is exhausting.

He takes his pills, juices, fruit, and a sweet roll. Then I do chores whilst he sits propped on a chair with a hassock, plenty of water, mags, a radio, etc. I mean I hustle. I get his lunch. Sometimes he falls to the floor. Often, I guess, because he is just frustrated and wants to walk. It takes three to get him up, or if only I'm here we do it alone! It has taken up to two or three hours as he crawls, hangs on to me, walker, etc.

Leisure? How do you spell it? I'd rather have an honest nine-to-five hard-work, straight-pay job any day! I must be candid even if I sound cruel. I'm not, really. . . . Not cruel. Just tired — bored — sad.

At this point I don't know what to do about Carlo. He is sixty-two and in robust health aside from the cruel MS. He is lucid, more an intellectual type — could I even put him in a nursing home had we the funds? How unhappy and rejected he'd be. Many people there (I've *seen*, with my mother) are certainly both physically and mentally incapable. Help to the individual home, I hear, is exorbitant and not so easy to come by.

Our younger daughter has set a wedding date. This is wonderful. Now — raising money for the reception.

*September 14, 1985.* The wedding was just beautiful, Carlo on a Foley catheter and walker. He and I were allowed to sit right at the side of the altar. The food a buffet dinner and a band played. At the end of what was enough for Carlo, three tall young men, all six foot or over, carried him down the steps to the car. At home alone, it took me from his chair in the living room to his bed about fifty minutes.

A physical therapist came out the two times allowed by Medicare. She said Carlo should be in a wheelchair but that if I were so determined to keep him ambulatory, I should put a heavy belt around his waist in order that I might handle him more efficiently from the waist, with less strain on my body. Sometimes my back or my leg hurts here or there and I guess that won't be getting any better so I am sitting with a heating pad on my knee as preventative medicine.

P.S. If someone comes, they'll mail this.

*February 22, 1986.* Life, as you are well aware by now, is not of such prime significance to me and were I to die this minute and rest six feet underground it would come none too soon.

I have the belt around Carlo's waist. This morning I fell over the catheter tube and it pulled out.

My sister-in-law and brother-in-law wanted me to take a vacation, too. Our older daugher said she would stay here, but Carlo won't allow either of the girls to bathe him or handle his Depends. He's been completely housebound since our daughter's wedding. We called various nursing homes. One wanted $62 per day, the best one costs $80. The home health care agencies indicated roughly the same thing, $72. My sister-in-law found a home that charged only $49.99, and I called them back two weeks before as they suggested and they were filled up. We were both disappointed. Carlo said it would be a nice vacation change for him — new scenery.

Carlo's disability checks are $697 monthly. His place of employment gives him a $157 monthly pension as long as he lives. We have some savings, and one large ($25,000) CD's interest helps. But rates are going down. His father left him the money so we were able to make a CD. Other, smaller ($7,000 and $10,000) CDs come from frugal savings. And we all worked so hard for it — Carlo, my dad and mom, Carlo's dad.

The kids have their own lives. Usually our daughters and sons-in-law try to help with getting things from stores and helping with chores here and there. But each lives far and the younger ones are out of work doing odd jobs. They try to help me by grass cutting, fixing things. Money is very tight for them and I've yet to see their home in the trailer court and they understandably are hurt. All four kids are being cheated!

The worst punishment is incarceration. That is the greatest argument against capital punishment. Incarceration with no parole, never a parole.

We should all live some before we die.

The visiting nurse that Medicare allows for an hour or so three times a week to help with the infection from the catheter suggested that I get a hospital bed.

*June 19, 1986.* Last week marked the first day of Carlo's confinement to the wheelchair.

Yesterday I took him to a geriatric specialist because I was worried about increasing sleepiness. Dozing, dozing, tired, tired! All tests prove he would be a healthy man were it not for the MS and the broken hip. The problem here — my back is aching me so much that I can't even sleep. Carlo is so heavy that it is completely a devastating thing just to attempt to get him from wheelchair to bed and vice versa. Today I called the visiting nurse and she doesn't think that even she could lift him, despite home aids. She told me I had "burnout" and they feel Carlo might have to go into a nursing home. I told her that he is only sixty-three. The doctor said he could live a normal longevity.

Years.

She said it might be me not living to be able to care for him and then his going into one anyway!

Where do I get the heart to put him in one? Where do I get the money? *Both* situations are driving me crazy.

The necessary heart may come when Carlo's medical team insists Liz give up — unless she collapses first. And the money?

Nursing homes cost between $20,000 and $40,000 a year. That's about $55 to $110 a day. Where could Liz get the money? Where could you get it?

From Medicare? No. Many Americans (79 percent, according to an American Association of Retired Persons poll taken in 1984) believe Medicare covers long-term nursing care, but it doesn't. This program was designed to deal with short-term acute care — mirroring the whole style of American medicine.

"If Medicare were to cover the costs of long-term care, we'd make Cap Weinberger look like a piker," says Representative Fortney Stark, chairman of the Ways and Means Subcommittee on Health, one of the three congressional committees handling Medicare and Medicaid.

From Blue Cross and Blue Shield? No again. Neither pays for long-term custodial care. (Though new plans are being tested.)

From another private insurance company? No again. Only about two dozen companies (see Appendix A) offer custodial care insurance and not many more than 200,000 Americans have bought it — annual premiums usually start high and rise steeply. Plans usually offer no more than $60 a day, which means the cheap end of nursing homes. Coverage seldom lasts beyond four years. Clauses concerning "existing conditions" often rule out immediate protection. (Nonetheless, it's an option to consider.)

From Medicaid? Only if you're poor. This federal plan to aid the poor requires needy middle-class families to become poor to get help. How poor? According to basic 1986 federal guidelines, assets can't exceed roughly $1,700 per individual or $2,550 per couple. Income can't exceed roughly $9,000 per couple. Now watch out. Don't take any of the numbers in this chapter for yourself. Specifics are given to help you conceptualize, to help you learn what questions you need to ask yourself and a lawyer: don't take any steps without consulting a lawyer versed in the Medicaid laws of your state. Basic guidelines can be dangerous. States administer the federal Medicaid program and each state modifies the guidelines, yielding a very complicated picture.

"It's difficult to generalize about Medicaid since the program varies greatly from state to state," warns Eugenie Mitchell, an attorney with the National Senior Citizens Law Center in Los Angeles. "In almost all cases, there are rules making some persons ineligible for Medicaid for a long time if they give away property for less than fair market value. Persons who anticipate that they will need Medicaid, expecially for nursing facility care, should consult with lawyers *before* making any property arrangements and before applying for Medicaid. This way, individuals can receive personalized advice. Otherwise, people may get rid of property which their state's Medicaid rules would have allowed them to keep, or they may end up with no Medicaid benefits for a long period as a penalty for having got rid of it. Local Legal Services lawyers provide free advice to persons whose income and assets are below certain levels. There are Legal Services offices to cover every area of the country. If your local Legal Services office can't handle your case for any reason, the office will usually be able to give you — if you ask — the names of private lawyers who are educated in Medicaid law. In this situation, a private lawyer's advice may well be worth paying for."

If a sick spouse qualifies for Medicaid, can the well spouse continue to possess the house and a car? Rulings vary state by state and a few wouldn't allow it. Depending on the state, a couple with Carlo's disability payments of $8,254 per year and his pension of $1,894 (totaling $10,148) would probably fall just above the line. They or couples like them in other states might make it onto Medicaid by special arrangements ("spending down") concerning income.

If Carlo qualified, Liz would lose the income she now lives on — Carlo's disability payments and his pension. These would go to his nursing home. In some states, a wife with no income is allowed several hundred dollars a month.

Getting Liz and Carlo's assets down to about $2,550 would mean losing their $45,000 in CDs and all but the face value of their life insurance. There's also a slim possibility, depending upon the state, of a wife or husband losing the house or half the house if the spouse qualifies for Medicaid. You can see why this process is referred to as spousal impoverishment.

"Right now we force people to impoverish themselves before they're helped, and that's just not right," says Representative Henry A. Waxman, chairman of the House Energy and Commerce Subcommittee on Health and Environment — another of those three committees that handle Medicaid and Medicare.

Will reform come?

Not in time for lots of us. If Carlo went into a nursing home now, Liz would escape her custodial slavery only for permanent poverty and dependency.

In a midwestern state, Leona refused to improverish herself. She and Everett had worked too hard and saved too carefully. When Everett was diagnosed as having Alzheimer's, Leona took care of him at home for nine years. She hung bells on the doors so she'd hear if he tried to leave in the night. For the last four years, she took him to an adult day care center twice a week at $15 a day. Then Everett suffered a stroke that paralyzed a leg and an arm. Leona's story demonstrates the frustration honest Americans feel in balancing a sense of justice with the demands of our medical insurance system. Simply finding out what's what is frustrating.

I didn't want Everett to go into a nursing home. But it took two people to move him and it was too hard, physically, for me. Medicare wouldn't pay for anyone to come in and help, not unless it was a professional nurse to give shots. For someone to help move a person or feed him or brush his teeth, you don't get any help. I had to put him in. I paid $2,000 a month for those first five and a half months — $11,500. Then I applied for Medicaid.

What took me so long was that I had to get rid of his assets, and if the spouse has too much they won't pay. In my state, you can have a house and its contents. Ours was in both names, but I moved it to mine anyway. The car is okay. I could keep my own Social Security, and my own pension. All his pension would go to the nursing home and all his Social Security, too. The big problem was that I couldn't find out exactly how much I was allowed to have. There were rumors that I couldn't have over $10,000. Was that the county? Or was that nationwide? The children and I, we couldn't even find out. We could never get the picture. So I didn't know how much I had to divest.

My son and daughter-in-law went in to try to find out what I'd have to do to qualify, and a social worker said that the patient can have only $1,500 in cash and a $1,500 burial fund — which you purchase at a mortuary. And $1,500 in life insurance. I had to get rid of all the insurance we'd been so careful to take out, except for $1,500 of it.

When some of my CDs matured, I took the cash and kept it in the freezer. My daughters were startled to see all that money sitting on the ice cubes. I gave them a few thousand each to buy me some CDs in their names.

Their biggest delay came in deciding about the life insurance. Everett had so much. He wanted to protect me. We didn't cash it in at first because after the stroke we thought he might die. Instead of surrendering the policies, I took out loans on them to pay for the nursing home. Then Everett stabilized and I paid back the loans and asked for surrender forms. I surrendered all but $1,500.

Then the day came. I went in shaking to the social services office with my checking account and my savings account and my CDs and my expenses by the month — all the bills. At the first meeting, the social services worker told me I should go back and do fix-ups on my house and so forth. She was nice. She said that if you need anything in your house that you've been waiting a long time for — a new furnace, a new floor, a new roof, you'd better do it now. You have to try to get your own money down in order to decrease the monthly allotment you have to pay. It was a big relief when we got out of there the first time. I was shaking. I couldn't function. The hardest part was I didn't know what to expect, economically or emotionally.

So I bought a new hot water heater and I got a kitchen floor and a new lawn mover. And I got myself a $1,500 burial trust, too. The funeral home invests the $1,500 in a CD for you, but they keep the records. All the interest is added. Any extra amounts for the funeral have to come out of your own pocket. They want to make sure the state won't be liable for burial monies.

I was more at ease the second time. After the meeting, the social worker took the figures to her supervisor and together they decided that I should pay $175 a month out of my own money to the nursing home. That meant that instead of paying $2,000 a month I just spend $900, which was what his pension and his Social Security and the $175 from my pension come to. I could appeal, but I didn't. I liked it a lot better than $2,000. When it finally came through, the decision, it was a big relief.

You give up so many things to set money aside and then suddenly you have to get rid of it. The anxiety of becoming eligible, that was difficult, too. The amount of money I had to pay out during those first months, a huge amount of money — I resented it. I couldn't have gone on paying privately. I would have depleted much of my assets. You don't know until you finally get there, that there's not a particular limit. If people know ahead of time, I suppose, they'd be able to figure out how to hide their money.

Leona's failure to report on her Medicaid application that she had transferred some of her assets to her children was illegal. If the Medicaid staff had found out, they could have delayed Everett's entry onto the Medicaid rolls for two years. That delay would have exhausted much of Leona's remaining assets. And in most states, if you are found to be lying on your Medicaid application, you may be in danger of having to pay back Medicaid benefits received or of facing prosecution.

One spouse to the nursing home, one spouse to the poorhouse? Something must be done to keep well spouses in the middle class without subterfuge. Something must be done to rescue well spouses from years and years of catheters and leg bags.

What?

Medicaid did pay $32 billion for nursing homes in 1984, or 40 percent of the nursing home bill. And this is up from $4.7 billion in 1970. The increasingly high tag strains Medicaid funds and limits other programs, such as those for the children of the poor and for poor pregnant mothers.

Who should pay for custodial care?

"Almost every elderly or disabled person is at risk of pauperization from long-term care in nursing homes or at home," says Senator Edward M. Kennedy, chairman of the Senate Committee on Labor and Human Resources — the third of the committees that deal with Medicaid and Medicare. "There is no question but that our society must address this problem if we are to fulfill the promise of Medicare: that our senior or disabled citizens can spend their well-earned retirements free from the fear that illness will deprive them or their spouses of a lifetime of savings."

Will the next few years bring an expanded Medicare program covering long-term custodial care for an additional annual premium of perhaps $800? (This is quite different from plans proposed in 1986 and 1987 to deal with "catastrophic illness", by closing gaps in acute or hospital coverage with an increased Medicare premium of $5 or $8 a month — or less for the poor and slightly more for the rich. "Catastrophic illness" in those proposals doesn't mean long-term illness: the gap being closed is not that of custodial care.) Will the years bring more private nursing home insurance with federal certification of companies to make sure they're viable? More in-home custodial care insurance? More individual medical accounts (IMAs) for custodial care, similar to IRAs? More continuing care communities for the well- and well-enough-to-do to buy into? The good news is that as the baby boomers reach middle age, demands for more complete health care coverage may force legislation.

Meanwhile you get to choose between slavery or penury.

# WHAT TO LOOK FOR IN A
# NURSING HOME

Dianne Goff-Debelle, a health care consultant and licensed nursing home administrator in Illinois, offers this list.

*Consider cultural needs.* Would your spouse be happier in a home with a particular religious or ethnic affiliation? Where a language other than English is spoken?

*Consider physical needs.* Does your wife or husband need physical therapy to increase the functioning of the large muscle groups? Someone who has had a stroke, for instance, will need a lot of physical therapy. Does your husband or wife need occupational therapy to maintain fine motor functions? Someone with Alzheimer's or a stroke may need this. Does your spouse need speech therapy to regain or increase verbal communication? Does she or he need a special diet? Radiation or chemotherapy? Special medical equipment? Which nursing home offers what your spouse needs?

*Will the doctor continue seeing the patient in the home?* Or will he recommend someone to follow?

*Is the home near enough for you to visit easily?*

*What are the home's financial admission criteria?* How will you meet the cost? Not all nursing homes, for instance, accept Medicaid.

*Meet with the admissions director.* At this meeting, you will discuss the needs of the resident and how they mesh with the home, as well as how you would finance residency. You might ask if the state license to operate and the administrator's license and the credentials of the medical director are all current. Find out if any special certifications have been given the home — such as one from the Joint Commission on Accreditation of Hospitals. It takes a lot of effort for a nursing home to be accredited. You may find the answers to some of these questions by looking at the certificates on the wall of the office. After the meeting, ask to tour the facility.

*What to notice on the tour.* In general, note cleanliness. Is the home as clean as you'd want your house to be? If it's a home that cares for the very disabled, there may be a urine odor. That's inescapable. In general, note the condition of furniture and equipment — is it torn? broken? dirty?

In the nursing unit, notice the appearance of the staff. Do they speak English? (Or whichever language the patient speaks?) How do the residents look? Are they appropriately dressed — in day clothes? Are they well groomed? Are there sufficient wheelchairs and other common equipment? Do there seem to be enough nurses and aides?

In the bedrooms, see if the walls and flooring are in good repair. How big are the bedrooms? How many beds in a room? If they're electric, do they work? Are there enough curtains or screens for privacy? How are the rooms heated? Air-conditioned? Do the windows open? Is there storage for personal belongings? A room for Alzheimer's patients should not have wood or inflammable furniture.

In the bath and tub or shower rooms, observe if there are grab rails. Curtains for privacy? Nonskid safety strips on the tub or on the floor of the shower? Do staff show concern for the privacy of residents?

Watch for evidence of the activity program. Is there a program posted? Is it being followed? If an activity is going on, how many residents are participating? What kind of resources does the home possess — movie or slide projector? VCR? phonograph? arts and crafts supplies? Are there individual games — such as cards, dominoes, mah jong, cribbage, backgammon? Do residents have to pay for activities? How many outings are planned during the year? And to where — ballpark? zoo? theater? Are there programs designed for various levels of abilities — for the disoriented, the disabled, and the alert?

In the kitchen area, see if meals are posted for general and individual diets. Is the menu varied? Is this kitchen as clean as yours? Does the food look appetizing?

Be aware of security. Are the fire exits and stairwells cluttered or clear for passage? Is the building secure in terms of the surrounding neighborhood? Are there alarms on exits and fire doors? Is there special security in the

Alzheimer's unit? People at certain stages of Alzheimer's walk constantly.

Inquire about the therapy department. Is the therapist a full-time employee or a consultant? If a consultant, what kind of daily program is offered? Who supervises it? Is there an extra charge for therapy? Is there a specific area allocated to it? Are there weights, pulleys, tables in the area? Hydrotherapy? Is there adaptive equipment, such as special cutlery so that patients who need it may feed themselves? Is it being used?

*Take time to decide.* Talk among the family and with the nursing home staff and with other members of the medical community about expectations and goals. It's important to make the right choice now.

———◈———

And the real end, the dying?

Rarely is the well spouse as desperate as the woman who told her husband's doctor: "Make it one cyanide, to go. If he won't take it, I will." Yet in the long chronics, a well spouse may not fear bereavement — he or she has already been bereaved. What's feared is that the other's breath may last into overwhelming pain, despair, or witlessness. Our years of ambivalence culminate in this final set of conflicting emotions, presented splendidly by David Young in his poem "Nine Deaths" (see Appendix B) for his wife, Chloe, dying unconscious and brain-damaged:

*I want to let you go. I want to keep you.*

During the span of chronic illness, a well spouse goes through preparatory grief and separation. "Anticipatory mourning is quite common," according to Dr. Richard Blacher (see Appendix B), former professor of psychiatry at Mount Sinai Hospital, New York. It "explains the frequent lack of a strong grief reaction in the survivors when death follows a prolonged illness." Grieving beforehand involves the gradual giving up of the dying person. If it happens too soon or too intensely, the well spouse feels isolated from the sick and then, perhaps, guilty after his death. Nonetheless, anticipatory grief is a natural, inescapable, and protective process.

Sally's story of bereavement bears an unusual element in Max's extreme denial. For seven years, they never even told his mother and father that Max was sick. Half a dozen years after his death, a beautifully groomed woman in her mid-forties sits in a living room in Berkeley. On the mantel over the fireplace is a photograph of a bearded, brown-eyed man in a ski parka. Outside, bright geraniums sit in clay pots on the patio. Inside, Sally leans gracefully against the soft, melon-colored pillows of the couch and reports in her low, confident voice how at twenty-three, she fell in love with Max, an architect, and married him. She, too, became an architect. They worked long hours. They did well. Things were wonderful.

"But what was the matter with Max's eyelid?" Sally leans a bit away from the pillows. "Had it always drooped like that?"

Max had myasthenia gravis, or MG. It affects either the ability to move limbs or the respiratory process, or both. They expected to be lucky, expected that Max would remit. Three years passed during which Max's illness was easy to conceal; then it got harder. They grew careful, watchful.

"If he got the flu, he could go into pulmonary arrest." Sally pulls away from the pillows and sits straight, without support. "Or into cardiac arrest. He could suffer brain damage." She presses a hand against her short, chic hair.

"Max's symptoms were erratic. It was hard to know what was what. A surgeon removed his thymus. How much medication to take? Max had to judge it. It was crazy. The symptoms of overdose resembled the symptoms of underdose! And that's not all. The medication actually brought on something new — asthma attacks. Did his gasping come from the MG or from the medicine? He could never be sure. I could never be sure."

Max kept going to work. Sally too.

"I didn't want to stay home from my job and take up a routine of nursing. He didn't want to, either. So we just kept on with our lives, as well as we could."

Sally handled his first asthma attack alone. "It was one morning a few weeks after the thymus operation, early in the morning up near the Russian River where our friends had lent us a house. I was sitting in a chair. From the bed, I heard labored breathing. I got him into the car. At the hospital the doctors all asked each other, 'Is it an asthma attack? Is it weakness from the myasthenia gravis?' They couldn't tell any better than we could. By then the attack was over."

Sally's voice grows tense, agitated. "I got to recognize his voice levels, gradations of his cough. I couldn't not notice. I was always waiting for him to cough or to finish coughing. With MG, that's how they can die, by respiratory failure. If his voice changed or thickened, if he coughed, I would tense up. I couldn't help it. I couldn't help listening. I was always sitting up straight and clutching onto something." Sally grabs onto the edge of the glass coffee table to demonstrate. "Alert, I was constantly alert and waiting. I couldn't relax."

She lets go of the table, leaving fingerprints, but remains tensely straight. "I would think to myself, there'll be *no end* of this. There'll be *no end*. I had fantasies of flight. I'd visit my sister in Seattle. At least I could talk about it with my sister. Max got more withdrawn and more isolated. He wouldn't talk about it. He simply did not think of himself as imminently dying.

"Finally I couldn't take it anymore and found a psychiatrist. I had to talk about it. He told me there's a lot of premourning that goes on. You mourn for and bury the marriage you had. You mourn for and bury the man you married. And then there you are. He's still alive. That's the way I felt. I loved Max. I hated what was happening to him, but it wasn't the marriage it had been."

"Somewhere in the sixth year I discovered that Max hadn't even made a will. He'd never bought a cemetery plot. When I found that out, I told him, 'If you don't plan for something, I can only assume you don't care how it's done.'

A week before he died I found a pamphlet on his bureau about wheelchair service at airports. At the last minute, he was admitting something was wrong. Up until then, he'd taken the plane with the rest of the boys and instead of rushing with them to catch the flight out from San Diego or St. Louis, he'd pretended he wanted to see the city. He'd rented a hotel room so he could stay over and rest up for the return flight."

Sally laces her fingers together and squeezes them.

"I got a draft form for a will and we filled it out. We couldn't talk about the end. We couldn't say 'what if.' So I made the decisions unilaterally. You make a lot of decisions by yourself, but you don't feel you're particularly in control of a lot of things.

"When Max went into a coma, I didn't know what to pray. I didn't pray. My brain gave me flashes of the future. That is, it flashed ahead to show me years of coma. It flashed ahead to show me him waking up with brain damage. I believed the doctors. I couldn't fool myself. Could I pray for him to live like that? I couldn't pray at all.

"I held off from choice. I had often wished that my life was not like it was, that the sickness had not happened to him, not happened to me. But when he was lying there in the coma, I found myself not praying, only thinking, 'This wasn't what I meant, God, when I said I didn't like the other.' I worried about having any contact with God. He seemed to be clumsy. Or hard of hearing."

With Max in a coma, Sally finally notified his parents.

"It was from a pay phone in the hospital lobby. There I stood, telling his mother how sick her only child was, that he was already in a coma. Of course, she couldn't believe it. She thought I hadn't been feeding him properly.

"After two weeks, he died. It was just this time of year, mid-July, five years ago. I always get sad this time of year."

Her eyes move to the photograph of the bearded, brown-eyed man. "That's Max. I usually visit my sister in July. The first year after he died, I flew up to visit her.

"There was a moment I remember at the airport. I got out of the plane and the air was beautiful. The scenery was beautiful. I rented a racy red car, a convertible with a radio, and I drove for an hour and a half along the Washington coast. The wind, the darkness of the pine trees, the great cliffs, the ocean view.

"Suddenly I realized that I was free from fear. It wasn't that I hadn't felt the loss. Or that I hadn't felt the grief, because I had. It was that I realized *nothing else can happen*. It had happened already. It was over. I was free of the fear. It was like the day the cast comes off your broken arm or leg. That's what you feel, the absence of fear. You've spent so long waiting for something bad to happen and then you realize it can't. Not that, anyway. Instead of feeling like this" — Sally unknots her fingers and grabs the coffee table again and her knuckles go white — "I finally let go."

She lets go of the table and sits back against the soft cushions, at last, and smiles.

"Did I tell you? I'm getting married next month."

Max died in a hospital. Forty families interviewed for a Consumers Union study researched and written by sociologist

Margaret Gold (see Appendix B) found hospices preferable for dying in certain respects: relationships with physicians, pain control, patient's body care, emotional support for patients and families, interaction with staff, and support during the hours of the death itself. Although hospitals tended to please families during the earlier stages of an illness, in later stages relatives sometimes felt too powerless against hospital attitudes and staff.

Of pain, one wife said, "When you see it, you pray for the end. . . . Please, God, just let him have peace." Hospices tended to give stronger medications and to keep the patient premedicated so analgesics never wore off.

On cleanliness, one family using a hospital had to resort to tipping service people in order to keep linens clean. "The more often we tipped, the better off we were."

On emotional support, one husband said that his wife had been bitter and withdrawn at home, but when she got into the hospice she wanted to be part of everything, was even carried in her bed to see a movie. Hospice volunteers relieved well husbands and wives and gave them a few hours away from the patient. Hospice workers helped family members voice their emotions. They gave privacy when needed, and comfort. And they were there for the dying. Would there be pain? fear? What awful sights would the family see? What awful sounds would they hear? Volunteers provided a helpful, knowledgeable presence, and when death came "they didn't herd us out — they let everybody in the family come in. They let us cry. They didn't try to shush us up because of the other patients."

Often we don't know what's out there in the new never-never land of technological life until too late. Francie didn't know that dialysis would depress Eric, or whether he would stay on it — 22 percent on dialysis opt to quit and die. Would doctors approve him for a kidney transplant? Would she herself hold together? Her voice over the phone began to sound small and whispery.

I got up today and found a note from Eric on the breakfast table. It said, "I won't be home tonight." That means he's telling me he's decided to . . . find a motel after his afternoon class and slit his wrists. He gets that way sometimes after the dialysis. I've called his department office and left a message. I've pulled him out of it before, but I'm so exhausted. I walk on such a tightrope. I've learned this — you can check out or you can endure. Those are the only choices.

We're talking about folding the magazine. My leave really affected its stability. I can't tell you how devastated that makes me feel.

Their two boys wanted to donate a kidney to Eric to increase the chances of a transplant working. Francie couldn't bear to have another family member cut up, nor did she want either child to lose 20 percent kidney function. Neither did Eric.

Eric has been interviewed and typed for a transplant. We'll have to wait two to six months. They say it's too bad we missed the Labor Day car accidents!

The magazine has folded.

That weekend, Eric panicked about the transplant.

He was pacing, banging his head, saying he wanted to jump out the bedroom window. I had to restrain him. He's afraid he'll go under and die during the operation. He started laughing compulsively. I told him I'd see him through.

What we do most of the time is simple survival. It's not heroic. What's heroic is when I go in to Eric when I'm worn out and when I reach down into the bottomless pit and find something else to say to bring him back. If I do that when I'd much rather go onto the patio and read, that's heroic.

Francie kept jogging in the park near her home and began to imagine flying off to Mexico. She also typed her résumé.

Still waiting for a Honda kidney — that's what they call them. Eric gets more disturbed every day. He's nuts. I'm so depleted all I think about is dying.

I'm so hostile, bitter, sad, scared, and exhausted I can't believe I'll make it through the weekend — much less the transplant, the posttransplant, the possible rejection, and the drug reactions. He's out of work. His disability hasn't begun. I'm out of work. What do we do for money? We've spent thousands on dialysis before they covered it.

Why are we put on earth? You shouldn't have to think thoughts like that after seventeen.

The phone is going to ring some night. I'm going to have to mobilize him and get him into the city. Then there will be three months of his not teaching and maybe he'll be loony on drugs again. When you write your book, don't water down the anger. That's what heroism really is — to go on loving them despite the anger. I'm mad all the time.

Francie invited some men who'd had successful transplants over to dinner and the evening convinced and relieved Eric. The next time the phone rang, her voice was almost back to how I remembered it in Chicago.

Yesterday just as I set Eric's lunch down in front of him, the phone rang. They got a kidney! He did fine. He's got a hose sewn in his neck. He actually told the anesthesiologist to go light, so he'd be awake for the football game! The man in the next bed got the other kidney. Macabre, huh?

It's such a relief to have him in the hospital. I don't have to sit on the bed and restrain him. He's not panicked anymore. He's not despairing.

The next week she began to slip.

Eric's so much better! He laughs, he jokes. From the first day, he was better. He said he could not possibly, could never, ever tell me how sick he had felt all that time — how full of toxins, how weak. He says he will never do dialysis again, he'd rather slit his wrists.

But now that it's over, I can't relax. I've learned two things. You survive. And you take it small. But I can't relax.

It's as though I've mourned him already. I don't know how to say this, but I mourned him before he died and then he didn't die. He's almost died several times these last eighteen months. And now he's resurrected. But I'm not sure I want him at home. Why should I get involved with him again? Expose myself to this all over again? He could reject any time. He's an attractive man. Let some other woman have him!

At the very most, we'll have some period of "now" to savor. Looking to any kind of future with Eric — I don't know. The kidney could last eight years. After that, he might need another. I've been avoiding what I feel because I don't want to feel it. I don't feel guilty about wanting to escape. I shouldn't feel guilty. It's just sad. It's a schizophrenic life. Something has happened to me. I have detached. I have mourned. I will have to renegotiate the whole thing.

Is he alive or is he dead? I can't help but think that without that stranger's kidney inside of him, he'd be dead. By nature's laws, dead. So maybe none of this happened. Maybe I made it all up? Sometimes it feels like that.

Come out here and visit me. I've got a job on a tourist magazine. We'll go to Hollywood and get discovered.

From a safe distance, technological medicine seems simple enough. Nobody wants to live a vegetable. Doctors will take care of it. Often they do, according to James H. Sammons, M.D., Executive Vice President of the American Medical Association. "For patients terminally ill with cancer, the patient usually makes the decision as to resuscitation or life-support with his or her family and their clergyman. . . . when hospitalized patients suffer cardiac arrest, hospital personnel make resuscitation efforts unless a 'Do Not Resuscitate' [DNR] order has been entered on the chart by the attending physician."

"I can think of no reason why a caring physician, who had discussed with a competent patient his or her beliefs about quality of life, would not follow those expressions in the event the patient loses capacity to express consent and the family or legal representative concurs in the patient's expressed desire," says Dr. Sammons.

But there are catches.

"It's easy to let a patient go," another doctor confides. "This talk of pulling the plug is innocent — we don't have to pull any plugs. All we have to do is just not to respond aggressively. It's very hard, you know, to stay alive on a ventilator or respirator. If there's an infection, a doctor simply doesn't give full doses of antibiotics. He simply waits before responding to any signs of trouble. That's all we have to do, really. If a doctor gets pulled into court he's either clumsy or the family has pressed him.

"The catch is, it has to be set up beforehand. The patient has to have talked with us. We don't need the living will for ourselves, we need it for the family. Say a man has had a heart episode and he's still out and we know there'll be severe brain damage when he wakes up. We talk to the family and say, 'Look, the prognosis is bad. There's brain damage. He wouldn't want to wake up. This is what he wants, he told me.' Then I pull out the living will and say, 'See what he gave me.'

"If the patient has discussed it with his family, the family may let him go. But if he hasn't, the loving family is apt to say, 'Save him!' So we save him. In a week he comes off the ventilator and it's clear he's severely brain-damaged. Then the family says, 'Okay, you were right. He wouldn't want to live like this. Do what you have to do.'

"But it's too late. He's off the respirator."

Saying no to extraordinary measures is one thing. Letting a wife or husband commit suicide is another. So's helping.

"She knew there would be pain at the end," the husband of a woman with leukemia says. "She asked me to get pills and, of course, I did."

It is a hard request to turn down.

"We're stockpiling Seconal," a couple reports, excitedly. "It's better than Nembutal because of its ten-year shelf life." Dosages barely whispered several years ago appear in best-sellers and on television interview shows, thanks partly to Derek Humphry's pioneering work (see Appendix B).

But the old joke holds: you have to be in perfect physical, mental, and spiritual shape to kill yourself. Once you're crippled or witless or installed in a hospital or nursing home, it's tough. An old man with advanced Parkinson's tries by biting his thermometer. A stroke victim tries to choke to death by swallowing his dentures. Both are "rescued" by staff.

"He keeps asking me for a gun," the wife of a paralyzed man reports. "I say no, never. He says he wants to die and will find a way to pull the trigger. I say no, never. I pray he'll be taken. But I could never shoot him. I just couldn't."

Could you handle the pills, but not the gun? If you're down to this debate, you're out of the great abstraction about whether it's right or wrong and into the small nagging questions. What if he drops the pills and you have to put them on his tongue? What if you get caught?

Judges interpret laws, not their own hearts. State law determines what happens if you help out in a suicide. In California, the law says it's a felony. In this liberal state, a new organization called Americans Against Human Suffering is trying to get a proposal on the 1988 ballot concerning the legality of aided suicide. A California judge recently gave partially paralyzed sixty-three-old Jay Ward McFadden three years' probation for holding a gun to the head of his wife Gladys, who had MS. She pulled the trigger.

In Connecticut, aided suicide is second degree manslaughter. In New York, it's second degree murder.

Laws change.

Hospital policies vary. Doctors may not respond aggressively when a patient is on a ventilator, but in the United States that's usually all a doctor does to help a patient die. In the Netherlands, doctors can legally inject the terminally ill who wish to die with appropriate drugs. It's called "the soft death." In the United States, it may or may not be possible just to order a feeding tube removed.

In 1983, a forty-six-year-old fireman, Paul Brophy, suffered an aneurysm and lay both comatose (joining ten thousand other Americans) and severely brain-damaged at New England Sinai Hospital. The hospital supplied him surgically with a gastric feeding tube. In 1984 his wife asked the hospital to take out the tube because her husband persisted in a vegetative state and she knew he would not want to live like that. The hospital refused. In 1985 Patricia Brophy, their five children, his ninety-one-year-old mother, and his seven brothers and sisters all petitioned release for Brophy from his mindless "life." A judge ruled it ethically inappropriate to take out the tube. It was already in place; it didn't constitute a burdensome procedure. In 1986 the Massachusetts state supreme court ruled 4 to 3 to let the tube be removed. New England Sinai Hospital still wouldn't allow it. Later in the year, the United States Supreme Court upheld the state ruling and the Brophys transferred Paul to the Emerson Hospital in Concord. There the feeding tube was finally removed, and days later Brophy's family stood around his bed — a grandchild climbed on it — to hold his hand, kiss his cheeks, and talk to him, as he managed to die.

The living but noncomatose death of Alzheimer's poses other problems. "We can't excactly take Grandma out and shoot her," a man explained to his daughter who recognized that her grandmother's life was not worth living. It takes five, ten, or fifteen years for an illness like Alzheimer's to make its host weak enough to die of infection. At what point would an Alzheimer's suicide be considered an aided suicide? A murder?

In Florida in 1985, seventy-six-year-old Roswell Gilbert brought his wife, Emily, home from the hospital where her chronic Alzheimer's did not qualify her for further stay and resumed washing and dressing her. In pain from osteoporosis, Emily wouldn't let her husband out of her sight. After three sleepless nights, he decided to go to a short condominum meeting for a break. She followed, calling, "I am so sick. I want to die." He took her back to the apartment and put two bullets through her head.

The court gave him twenty-five years for first degree murder with no parole. (He was a "cool" witness; McFadden wept in court.) When the Florida appeals court confirmed the sentence in 1986 on the grounds of its clear legal mandate, the opinion nonetheless held a qualifier slanted to legislators:

> Whether such sentences should somehow be moderated so as to allow a modicum of discretion and whether they should allow distinctions to be made in sentencing between different kinds of wrongdoers, for instance, between a hired gangster killer and one, however misguided, who kills for love or mercy, are all questions which, under our system, must be decided by the legislature and not by the judicial branch.

Until then, what's legal?

Living wills, though they're hardly foolproof.

"It's getting easier to get a respirator turned off it you have a living will," says Mrs. A-J Levinson, executive director of Concern for Dying, a New York–based organization that distributes living wills. "Doctors and hospitals are more consistently willing to do it. They're also more willing to write DNR orders. The sticky issue now is the feeding tube. Some people view artificial feeding as a medical treatment and some do not. It is very clear," continues Levinson, "and it has been upheld in many courts that there is a constitutional right to privacy and a common law right to bodily self-determination — i.e., any competent adult may refuse any form of medical treatment at any time. It is equally clear in law that an incompetent person cannot be denied the rights of a competent person. The only point at issue is how an incompetent person exercises the right. The best way is to sign a Durable Power of Attorney while competent, naming someone else to make life or death decisions for you if you become mentally incompetent and to give that person specific instructions in a living will."

Act now.

Plenty of material exists on death, dying, actual bereavement. At the final crisis, we are usually aided by the support and comfort of the acute emotions — friends and family join round about us. We have mourned the marriage that was, the person that was, the future that was to be. We've endured the chronic emotions. We stuck. No acknowledgment from strangers matters now — we know what it was, we know what it took. We did it. We forgive ourselves for where we failed. We're ready. We know we'll mourn, that anticipatory mourning isn't all there is to it. Hopefully, we've made the most of what was left and planted the seeds of a survivor's life. Now time that stopped at diagnosis and split into his time and her time flows back into one time — it's over.

---

# FINAL ARRANGEMENTS TO MAKE IT EASIER LATER

1. *Talk about the future with your spouse.* If yours won't or can't talk, seek informed friends.

2. *Attend at least one meeting of a support group concerned with your spouse's illness.* You'll find people who know what services you're entitled to and which are actually available nearby. The grapevine remains a superb source of practical knowledge and a good early warning system.

3. *Start files.* Clip articles on Medicare, Medicaid, the Veterans Administration (if applicable), and area agencies, including those for the aging — even if you're younger. The aging and the disabled form a single cluster.

4. *Understand Medicare Medical Insurance (Title 18 of the Social Security Act).* In general, Medicare Part A covers short-term hospitalization and Part B covers physicians and certain services. Anyone who has received Social Security disability payments for two years is eligible, despite age. Medicare also covers (partially, and depending on your plan) up to one hundred days in a nursing home — but only if a patient coming from a three-day or longer hospital stay is too weak for home care. And, if a physician requests it, Medicare will send a nurse home three times a week for several weeks to give drugs or to

change dressings; it will provide some physical and speech therapy for those unable to leave home without help. Medicare may pay for five days of respite care in a nursing home. Medicare is currently the largest sponsor of home care, paying out $1.7 million in 1984, a sum that constituted but 2 percent of Medicare's massive budget.

To find out more, call the local Social Security Administration. As mentioned earlier, look in the white pages of your phone book under the United States Government listings, and within them under the Health and Human Services Department and record the name of anyone who talks with you at length.

5. *Understand Medicaid Medical Insurance (Title 19 of the Social Security Act).* Are you and your spouse poor enough to qualify for Medicaid? To find out, talk with a lawyer well versed in the Medicaid laws of your state. Even if you can get onto the Medicaid rolls, it isn't a perfect system. If Medicaid pays for a pair of glasses (not all states offer this) for your spouse and he drops them three days later, he may have to wait a while for another pair. If your spouse loses fifty pounds and her new dentures (not all states allow dentures) don't fit, she, too, may have to wait. But basic custodial care will be provided. Depending on the state, Medicaid also pays for adult day care (including transportation) and for a one- or two-week respite in a hospital so that the family can get a break.

To find out your state's formal asset and income limits, call a local Medicaid office. How do you find the number? It's not always easy. Look in the white pages under state listings. Try the Department of Public Welfare, the Department of Medical Assistance, the Department of Human Services, the Department of Social Services, the Department of Human Resources, the Department of Welfare, or the Department of Health. In some states, county listings yield the right offices. If you get too frustrated, call your local library and ask for the reference librarian. She may look in the *National Directory of State Agencies* to find a number for you. Or you could look for an Information and Referral Service number under your town's Social Service Agency listing.

When you get someone from a Medicaid office on the phone, don't say, "My husband is disabled and I need to look ahead. Do I qualify for Medicaid?" The answer would probably be "Tell me what you have in assets and income and I'll set you up for an intake procedure." Instead, say, "What are the state's income and asset levels for Medicaid? Does the house need to be in the well spouse's name? Does the car? Do the assets include life insurance?" This is all public information and you're entitled to it.

What you hear formally by phone may give you either too rosy or too grim a picture. Let's look at Massachusetts, a lenient state — along with California and New York. During the second half of 1986, a family of four in Massachusetts could not receive Medicaid if they had an income greater than $741 a month ($8,892 annually) or assets beyond $2,000 for the applicant and $1,000 for the spouse. Each child could hold assets of $100. The well spouse could keep a house and a not-too-spiffy car.

Should a resident with a sick spouse act? Begin to divest? How fast? How slowly? If investigators suspect that property has been tranferred to meet qualification levels, they might possibly check back further than the standard two years recited by phone. Yet this Massachusetts Realtor who got her advice from non-Medicaid lawyers may be moving too slowly:

> My lawyers urged me to put the house in my children's name in a living trust and to wait five years. It's been four and a half now and I'm half dead. I'm waiting until my husband gets an infection again and goes into the hospital. When he's there, I'll tell them that I can't do the nursing anymore. They'll assign him to whatever nursing home within a fifty-mile radius has space. That could make a long drive, but I didn't want to lose my house.

Here's what to do. Talk to a lawyer. And not just any lawyer. Follow Eugenie Mitchell's advice. Call your Legal Aid office (first few pages of the phone book or under the town's agency on aging or within the Human Services entries). Ask what the limits are for free advice. If they are too low for you, ask them to recommend a lawyer versed in your state's Medicaid laws.

The knowledgeable lawyer will discuss whether you can qualify for Medicaid without violating rulings that prohibit giving assets away. Depending on the state, the lawyer may suggest you divide your assets and start to hold property not jointly but separately — half and half. The lawyer might mention ways of spending down, buying a life insurance policy or paying for in-home nursing care and possibly home improvement out of the sick spouse's separated assets. The lawyer may explain that after a sick spouse has been in a nursing home for six months (this period may soon change), the well spouse may begin to possess more assets.

6. *Understand Supplemental Security Income (Title 20 of the Social Security Act).* SSI is a joint federal and state effort designed to help the severely impaired, the blind, and the very old. It provides financial aid for the unemployed poor who don't have sufficient work history to qualify for Social Security Disability. Anyone on SSI qualifies for Medicaid.

7. *Consider a continuing care community.* Could you afford one? About 150,000 Americans (though the number increases daily) have bought into these, but many communities don't accept people already evidencing illness.

8. *Consider private custodial care insurance.* Ask your own insurance agent what's available. See also Appendix A for some companies offering partial coverage for nursing home care and for some experimental programs covering partial in-home care. Be careful of medigap insurances because they usually don't offer nursing home coverage and very little, if any, home care coverage.

9. *Consider adult day care.* Would this help enough? For the mentally ill and those with organic brain syndromes (such as Alzheimer's), it may be the answer — at least for a third of the day. Churches, nursing homes, and private concerns offer such centers. Without Medicaid, the daily cost may run from about $20 to $25, not including transporation. But how would you manage from, say, 3 P.M. to 9 A.M.? And how would you transport a paralyzed spouse?

To find a center, check the yellow pages of the phone book under Day Care, Adult. Or check the first few pages of the book (or the blue pages, if you have them) for elderly services, including your area agency on aging.

10. *Consider respite care in a medical facility.* Can you get by with just a week or two off a year? This fast-growing alternative gives the well spouse a short but intense break

and the sick spouse a dramatic change. Medicaid may pay for five days of respite, although some conditions are excluded. Without subsidy, the cost runs to about $100 a day. For more information, call the local chapter of the foundation associated with your spouse's illness or area agencies on aging — look under county listings, or in the very front of the phone book.

11. *Consider in-home care.* Can you afford it? The well spouse pays for most home aid, if he or she can find anyone to do the work. Visiting nurses may charge $12 to $14 an hour and many nurses won't even do this custodial work — it's too hard. Agency nurses' aides may charge $7 to $8, although they keep only about $4 for themselves. Check local nursing agencies to find out what they offer and if they handle your kind of case. See the front pages of the phone book for county listings for area agencies on aging. Read about home nursing (see Appendix B, Murphy).

12. *Make a will.* One-third of Americans die intestate. Most states award a third or a half of the estate to the spouse and two-thirds or a half to the children. Remake earlier wills filed in a state you no longer inhabit. If your spouse won't discuss wills, you may want to follow Sally's example and draw them up yourself. Sally used a simple form available at certain stationery stores and got it notarized. Each state has its own forms. These are valid, but of course there's always the problem that you may make costly mistakes or overlook advantages a lawyer could suggest. Lawyers' fees for making a will tend to run around $150 for a modest estate.

13. *If you possess more than roughly $600,000, consider an estate planner* (in a community property state, make that $1,200,000). You may possess much more than you think. An estate includes stocks, bonds, real estate, savings and checking accounts, household furnishings, cars, jewelry, collectibles, proceeds from life insurance policies, annuities, retirement benefits — including IRAs, profit sharing, and stock purchase plans, and all assets over which you hold general power of appointment. To the first session, bring complete lists of possessions and of who owns what, listing beneficiaries and information about which spouse has the right to change beneficiaries.

An estate planner will "look at your assets and liabilities and try to position them in the right entities to minimize death or transfer taxes to the government," as estate planner and certified public accountant Jimmy Averitt of Dallas puts it. Commercial banks have offered estate planning for some time and so, since 1982, have certain savings banks. Costing perhaps $100 a session, meetings with an estate planner yield ideas for protecting your estate from unnecessary taxation, as well as the delays and costs of probate. If you plan to pay out of pocket for the nursing home of a sick spouse, ask about appropriate trusts. You need roughly half a million in principal to yield $40,000 a year for a nursing home. When the plan is complete, a lawyer draws the will.

A number of attorneys, insurance salesmen, accountants, and just plain free-lancers plan estates, too. Some are wonderful; some not. Jimmy Averitt suggests calling the state board of public accountancy or the state bar association to check. Or simply go to the trust department of a major bank. If you fear your spouse may become mentally incompetent, if might be wise to choose an estate planner who is an attorney.

14. *Estimate this: What will you live on?* After your own retirement? If your spouse dies? goes into a nursing home? What would your spouse live on if you died?

15. *Figure out when you should open talks with a lawyer.* To find out if you qualify for Medicaid? To make a will? To declare someone mentally incompetent? To sign two Durable Powers of Attorney assuring that if either of you loses your marbles, the other can make decisions? Steps may interrelate. Think it through. Ask how to provide for your spouse if you die first. How to make it clear that a trust for your spouse should be considered as supplemental to SSI or Medicaid support. (Leaving money to a sick spouse may disqualify him or her from federal aid until the assets are gone.) Can you leave money to a relative or friend for a few luxuries or necessities for the sick spouse?

16. *What about divorce?* Some couples go past separation of assets to full divorce in order to qualify for Medicaid or veterans benefits without impoverishing the well spouse.

17. *Consider novel solutions for custodial care.* After you've gathered sufficient information, sit down and talk with

whatever friends, family, and advisers surface. Could you provide room and board to a student who would give custodial care in return? Could you buy a two-family house and trade an apartment for nursing care? How about group housing?

If nothing works, you might start your own group of custodial care givers. Why not? Because it takes a person with some time on her hands and some know-how about public agencies, especially if you intend to seek funds. It's not chance that Women Who Care got started in Marin County, one of the wealthiest residential areas in the country. But this last resort is worth a shot. Write or call model groups (see Appendix A) for advice.

18. *Talk with each other about dying.* Be very clear about extraordinary measures. It isn't easy to say "no" to the interns when they come rushing some night to ask, "Shall we resuscitate?" If you don't want resuscitation, or gastric tubes, or ventilators, practice saying no with each other and for each other ahead of time. Voice your decisions to your doctors.

19. *File living wills with your doctors.* To acquire wills, contact the Hemlock Society or Concern for Dying or the Older Women's League (OWL) (see Appendix A). It's safest to fill out a living will specific to your own state and to initial it every year or so — how about Memorial Day? This makes it clear that yours is a longstanding wish. Be specific about which measures you want to reject — the living will will ask for your choices — about resuscitation, ventilator use, and gastric tube. Ask these organizations for Durable Power of Attorney forms as well, and state these same choices on them. You might also ask your hospital how seriously patients' directives are taken.

20. *If suicide is an option, educate yourself.* Consult the Hemlock Society (see Appendix A).

22. *Get funeral arrangements out of the way.* The average full (that means the body is in the room) funeral runs between $2,500 and $3,000, although it's impossible to say exactly: cemeteries charge varying amounts to open plots; some cemeteries sell their own grave liners and some don't. Simpler cremations with a memorial service (the body is not in the room) may run from $1,000 to $1,500 cheaper, depending on what you want for services. You

can choose arrangements now and not pay until later. Or you can prepay. If you prepay, the funeral director is obliged by law to invest the money and use the interest toward later charges (cemetery charges, for instance) that may inflate before you die. If you feel you need to be armed before entering the funeral parlor, write the National Funeral Directors Association for pamphlets and guidelines; OWL's pamphlet on funeral arrangements is tidy, too (see Appendix A).

23. *Keep track of hospice care in your area.* Write the National Hospice Organization (see Appendix A) and ask what in-home, in-hospital, and in-hospice services exist in your area. Hospice care came to this country in 1974. A hospice is not so much a place as a concept of care designed for patients who do not expect to live longer than a few weeks or months. Hospice affirms dying as a normal process and seeks not to hasten nor to delay it but to make it as pain-free and as full of loving attention as possible. If you're eligible for Medicare Part A, a hospice death is covered — so long as you die in 210 days (and so long as the hospice is Medicare approved).

Much of the hospice care offered is given at home. Medicare attempts to cover home nurses, aides, drugs, respite, and counseling for the family, but find out exactly what you would be entitled to. Is it really enough? In-hospice care may take place in special homelike institutions with curtains and stuffed chairs. It may also be offered in local hospitals, since many of them provide a few hospice rooms or beds.

"Strange," the small, alert woman in the hospice bed said to her visitor. "I'm ending my life with Kafka." Her fingers rested on the new biography of the surrealist writer. A tube ran into her nose.

"I began my adult life with Kafka, in college. But I've had such a simple life, such a happy life, such a sane life. Why Kafka? It's strange."

Outside her window an iron stork stood over the maternity wing.

She smiled. "This morning I told my daughter what I wanted for my last breakfast — a croissant and a coffee, light. You know, when it came, I couldn't eat it."

The visitor smiled back. So this is the way it is.

"Oh, could you do something? I borrowed a book from the library and I'm afraid it's . . . overdue. I've had it on my list of things to tend to, but now I wonder . . . could you . . . ?"

"Sure. I'll return it."

She handed the visitor a book, and the next day she moved from total consciousness into a coma, and the day after that she died.

We don't always get to finish our lists.

# Chapter 21
# Everything in Its Place

You can see Los Angeles from the sky, a nub of land nosing out into the blue sea with its tiny white waves. Streets and boulevards crisscross the nub and then I am on land and Francie is waving.

"L.A.X.," she calls out in her up-front way, "you should have flown to Burbank!" How casually chic she looks with her gray legging pants and her baggy black sweater, her silver earrings, her sensual face lined now. Was I always taller? It's been seven years since Chicago.

We find the car in a highrise full of cars and then she is jumping lanes and talking animatedly. "I've got people coming over tonight. You'll meet the intellectual community of Pasadena. I'm sorry it's tonight but there was no other . . ."

The great sprawl of the city, the tall palms that are real, not part of a movie set. It looks as tangled out there as the Bronx and Staten Island rolled into one, but southern, almost Mediterranean. We come off the highways and onto streets full of Spanish architecture.

"That's the San Gabriels, but you can't see them today." Houses turn to redwoods and they're spaced about as far apart as on our street in Highfield; the grass is so much greener.

"All watered," Francie confesses. "Think of it as imported grass."

"And that?"

"Orange trees, can't you tell?" She pulls up beside a redwood house with a kelly green lawn and lemon trees, yes, lemon trees, in front. "Eric's home. We'll talk later."

A big graying, dark-haired man whose face is swollen with prednisone opens the door.

"Hello, Maggie," he extends his right hand. He takes the suitcase out of my hand. He kisses Francie and he shuts the door; the hall seems faintly Japanese. Their boys are off, one hiking in Scotland, the other waiting tables in La Jolla.

"What do you think of Los Angeles?" In the kitchen with its blue and white and copper, Eric opens a bottle of wine with the strength and control it takes to operate a corkscrew.

This is a sick man? You're kidding.

Of course, it's exactly what Francie means. You don't know. Eric could reject his cadaver kidney tomorrow. He could bleed internally tonight. He could die.

In the morning, Eric drives to the university and Francie and I walk in the Arroyo Secco at the foot of the San Gabriels. She tells me how she fell apart after the transplant.

"I knew the voices were inside my head. I knew I wasn't really going crazy, but I felt this tingling all over. I thought I had a brain tumor. My doctor asked if the tingling were in both hands and when I said yes, he said relax, it's not a tumor. Just in my head. I knew that. I went back into therapy. I had to sort out the voices, even though they were my own. They were all the parts of myself that I couldn't have, couldn't be, couldn't do, for those eighteen months when Eric was in danger. All the things I couldn't say. Now I'm better. But, of course, he'll always be in danger. We're into the age brackets where you can pick up the phone and expect bad news. I'm not ready. It was too fast."

We stand in what should be golden California and it's dry, with an aged smell to the land, like a good wine.

"I lost so much in a year and half. I didn't know who I was. Who am I? It was as if I'd committed spiritual suicide without knowing it. I didn't think I could get together with Eric again. After all, he'd been living such an excruciatingly separate life from mine. There was such a gulf. I was lonelier than if I'd never married. To survive, I'd had to detach, split off. I had to hold onto the parts of me that were separate from him. I was afraid that the minute I reconnected with him, he could die all over again. I began to understand why he puts his worst feelings aside. You have to live *as though* you're going to live."

That night Eric drives us to dinner. He lets us off at the door and parks the car. He leads the way to the table. He orders the sushi. I can't begin to explain to Francie how different things are at my house.

The next day Francie and I drive through downtown, or really the various downtowns, to the square near the *Times Mirror* with its skyscrapers. The great and marvelous mix of Hispanics and whites and Asians reminds me of New York, as does all of Los Angeles with its glorious messy vitality. With all that sun, the poorer parts lack the sometimes sinister threat of New York's manmade canyons.

And then we are driving out to the beach house at Malibu that a student of Francie's from her magazine workshop has lent her. We walk along the cliffs in our straw hats and jeans. We climb down to sand and walk.

"I got better out here." Francie walks in the foam and I in the damp, darkened sand, listening to the waves echo against the cliff wall. We are in the prime of life. We look younger than our years. We were struck at the height of our powers. We still feel the power and the desire for life, if only we could be freed to concentration.

"From now on," Francie says, "I'm going to put my work first. That's my top priority. The old staff is talking about getting up a new magazine."

I look out at the great ocean whose history I scarcely know. There's so much to know and do in life!

At the airport, I realize Francie has left me. She has returned to the well world. Suddenly I feel abandoned on the shore of a dark lake.

"Don't worry." She hands me my plastic bag filled with shells and bits of palmetto and hibiscus. "I'll be back. Any minute. I can't tell when, but I'll be back."

"Have fun!" she calls as I walk under the curved arch and make it blip.

"Fun!" I call back as I take off my silver bracelets to pass through again.

"Fun!" She's far away now.

In San Diego, I looked out over the perfect bay from the Cabrillo Monument. In San Francisco, I walked on the spit of land high over the dainty, curling Japanese ocean at Point Reyes. It was wonderful to be away. My work has taken me from home before, but never so long. For two weeks I walked at my own pace and lived in my own time frame — the high prime.

In the plane over Chicago, I couldn't eat any lunch: I didn't want to go home.

Ted had the front porch light on and was walking slowly into the hall. When we embraced, I remembered to be careful of his fragility. We sat at the dining table. He'd fallen and bled from the nose on the day I'd visited the San Diego Zoo but decided not to tell me. Debbie rushed in from downtown with a friend to say hello and rushed out again. Seth had filled the house with food and would be back at about eleven from his telephoning job. I told Ted California. He looked the same, patient, curious, kindly. Yet as we spoke, my sense of the healthy life drained slowly away. Why was I so tan?

Tim and Eileen visited that weekend and we drove to the top of a mountain with a 360-degree view. I stood in a basement of the summit house waiting to help Ted up the stairs when he came out of the bathroom. Wearing Edwardian straw hats, Tim and Eileen walked out over rocks and uneven terrain to a grassy ledge. They moved in a dappled green light over the hill and out of sight. They were probably standing at the place where you can see into three states at once. When they came back into view, they walked slowly toward me. They walked in such a leisurely way together — not quite but almost as far into their forties as Ted and I had been when we got the news. Graceful people, how well they walked together, their legs moving to the same beat, their hips. They were holding hands and the sun dappled them again through trees. Such simple blessings, so taken for granted, so irreplaceable. They saw me and I climbed a few steps out of the shadowed archway, still near enough to hear Ted if he needed me.

"Was it hard to leave Ted?" Tim asked in the beautiful light.

"No." I stuck my hands into my pockets of my white skirt. "It was hard to come back."

They were silent, shocked. I'd forgotten that they didn't speak my language. There was no time to explain. It doesn't mean I don't love Ted. It means I, too, would like to walk to the ledge to see the view. But with Ted, I can't. Ted can't. He isn't feeling well and needs to start home as soon as possible. I've been two whole weeks free of this terrible illness, which Ted can't ever get free of except in dreams, and you better believe that it was wonderful. Imagine, if Ted could be free of it for two weeks?

"You're so tan! And you look taller, lighter on your feet!" Thea met me the next morning at the pool where she gives me her sense of the good in life. At her kitchen table, Nellie delivers me her knowledge of the beautiful. At an Italian restaurant, Nick reminds me of the true: that unless he gets a National Endowment or a Guggenheim, he'll be forced to stop his series of watercolors. Jane called from New York to say she might take a big job offered her in Houston even though Patrick doesn't want to leave Horace Mann. Sid and Mim looked wonderful; Andrew is taking a summer course at MIT and Gracie is dancing in the Balanchine summer school. And Trisha called to say her son has leukemia. He's fifteen. On his bald skull, she says, they've painted a red cross for their radiation nozzles.

No one escapes. In the fourteen months that I have been writing this book, one friend has gotten a brain tumor. Two have ended marriages. One's son has dropped out of college and into drugs. One's daughter is nine months pregnant with twins and one of them has spina bifida. A former colleague has died of lung cancer. In the fifties, our friends have caught up with us. We married late. We aged early. Our green years were short. My mother loses daily to her renal failure. Life, on the downside, is a terminal illness.

There's a widespread folktale in which a woman has suffered some great sorrow — it differs according to which version of the tale — and is told to bake or boil such-and-such, in a pot or cauldron that has never been used to cook a meal for mourning. She must borrow the pot from neighbors. Of course, no neighbor possesses such a pot. The woman finds that loss visits everyone.

And that's only individual sorrow. The large-scale and malevolent disasters put these in shadow: war, earthquake, poverty. We must see our children in terms of all the world's children — the newborn daughters of the young soldiers who died in the Thirty Years War, the young sons of every city block that is poor in goods or poor in spirit. The point is to be able to go on with some delight after we have passed beyond the innocence of the good, undamaged years. Because there are the good years and then the bad years and then the years that, because they're not so bad, are sometimes wonderful.

My father used to tell me the story of a man and wife whose five children were killed in an earthquake and flood when the parents were temporarily out of the house. The couple mourned for a long time, and then they went out and built a new house and turned it into an orphanage for the countryside. They raised about twenty children in it. How I hated that story. The random violence of it. The tackiness of that relentless usefulness. Everything, I hated it all. When I grew up and had my own children, I hated it more. How could my father have believed that those twenty other children replaced the five beloved ones? Now that I am in the prime of life, I finally understand the story.

We grow slowly. After one of those work weekends when I visited my mother and came home to the lawn and the bills and the squabbles, I sat at night depleted in the living room. Seth's stereo played upstairs. Ted slept.

Debbie ran noiselessly downstairs, on her way to town to meet friends. Although I knew she'd prefer to be alone, I told her I wanted to walk her to the corner. We went into the darkness, under trees black against the sky. Porch lights burned along the street, television sets glowed palely beyond windows, dogs roamed the dark lawns. It was silent, too silent.

"Aren't you wearing shoes?"

"Oh, Mom!"

A fight. Debbie went angrily back for shoes before we resumed walking, her shoes untied: schlump, schlump, schlump.

"I'm cutting through here." She tried to dump me by taking a shortcut across a lawn to the back path that runs its shadowy way down a hill into town.

"I'll walk you to the top of the path." I hung on. I'd just relax, say nothing, be. Anything was better than the house. We reached the top of the dark, leafy passageway. Long ago, we'd skied down here to buy a candy bar. In the summer dark, Debbie turned to me and flung her arms around me, sobbing.

"Oh, Mom, how can you stand it? Your mother is dying and your husband is falling apart and you try . . . you try every day. I love you."

"Thank you," I told her, crying, too, as I hugged her. "I love you. Go and have some fun."

Off she went. She was growing! She didn't see me as just her mother anymore or Ted as just her father. She saw herself as a woman, her life as a woman ahead; she saw my life. And I was growing, too. I'd kept my mouth shut at the right time and opened it at the right time.

It was Nick's and Claire's and Nellie's night to cook and they were doing curried chicken in the kitchen. Ted looked white when I got home over the ice from the office.

"How was the writers' meeting?"

"I didn't go." He sat thin and insubstantial in the living room, retreating from the heat of the kitchen.

"Too slippery?" I took off my gloves and sat beside him on the dark couch. No fire in the fireplace, we know now that's for spring and fall. The living room seemed dim and cold, curtains drawn, lights low.

"I couldn't get my new coat on." Ted sat with his head down. He'd skipped first grade. The second-grade teacher had had to help him, only him, with the zipper of his snowsuit. "My hands wouldn't go."

"Oh, Teddie. I'm sorry."

"And then Ann came to get me to drive to the meeting, but it was too slippery to get to the car."

"Awful. But it's awful out there."

Thea and her husband, Charles, rang the doorbell. It was time to eat. Nick had brought his VCR and a video of *City Lights*. We all seven sat wrapped in blankets watching.

In bed, with our comforters pulled high, I remembered the women and men I'd talked to for this book. How Steve in Maine had said that until Jerilyn could accept her blindness, he couldn't, and that this had made it hard for him. How Max had never even told his parents about his myasthenia gravis and didn't want Sally to tell anyone. No wonder we feel invisible. We really can't deal with the disease until they do, can't fully mourn and begin to grow again around the devastation. I felt terribly sad.

"I'm sad," I said to Ted.

There was a silence and I thought of friends. Any one of them would have instantly asked why.

Finally the words came from Ted. "What about?"

"Your coat. The ice. It's very sad."

"Don't think about it." He joined in quickly then. "Think about a yard of green grass growing in Saudi Arabia or the beautiful colors in the dome of the Taj Mahal."

Instead, I thought of the women and men I'd interviewed. "I don't want to. I want to feel that I'm sad. It's real. It's how I feel. It won't kill me. I want to feel it. I want to feel it with you."

No reply.

Okay. I'd go to sleep. At least I'd said it. We may not exist together, but I won't let Ted take my emotions away from me, even if he doesn't care to share them.

Twenty minutes later, he spoke into the darkness. "I see what you mean. I see what I do. You said you were sad and I deflected it. But I can't let myself feel sad, I'll break apart. I'll collapse entirely."

"You've been saying that for years. It's destroying you."

"That's ridiculous! What's destroying me is MS!"

"MS is destroying your body. Your emotions are still your own. You could still have them."

"Maybe," he said, his voice breaking. "Maybe when the stress is off and you get your book in, I'll take a week and cry."

"That's my vacation week!"

"Well, I can't do it before!"

"Okay, good, do it then."

I lay there thinking something was missing. I'd missed something vital. What was it? Oh, yes, that he could cry by himself! He didn't need me for every tear!

Then I heard him. Just a few tears, no real sounds, but I knew. I didn't reach out. I didn't comfort him. I lay as if asleep. It was wonderful. He was doing it alone. Later, we could do it together.

Looking in a drawer for something for Ted's fifty-fifth birthday party, I found Seth's eighth-grade pictures. There he sits against the false shimmering background in his red plaid shirt, his dark hair curling and his eyes appraising the camera. He's smiling an emerging grown-up's smile: not a kid grin, not an adolescent's refusal, but an attempt at compromise. It hadn't worked. His smile had the same false shimmer as the photographer's background. But there he is again at thirteen trying to become — once in large size, twelve times in wallet.

I miss my lost children. I can hardly remember them during the years of my economic crisis. But most mothers feel this way as the family disassembles. And all marriages have tough spots, dependencies. The marriage with chronic illness is just more so. All lives have disappointments and losses, the well spouse's are just harder to remedy. All those "more so's" and "harders" add up into a pattern now familiar.

Last winter Francie and I sent letters that crossed. We'd each enclosed the same newsclipping and actually underlined the same words. It was an interview with the mother of Marilyn Klinghoffer — whose husband, Leon, was killed by terrorists during a Mediterranean cruise. Rose Windwehr told reporters, "I'm strong. You know how you get strong? You meet each situation as it comes. Over a lifetime all these situations add up, one after another. And then you're strong and old." Francie and I had each underlined the last four words.

I hope you will find a friend like Francie with whom to speak the pidgin of well-spouse-ese. I hope your friend has a sense of humor, even if it's black humor. One of Francie's letters hangs over my desk. It comes from the time when she and Eric were waiting for a dying man's kidney. In it she's typed out a poem from a book about living happily with kidney failure. I won't quote the poem. The woman who wrote it doesn't deserve such flack from Francie and me, not at all, not one bit. So I'll write a new one, along the same lines.

> WAITING FOR A TRANSPLANT
> When you have a kidney failing
> You must try not to be blue.
> Just use the time more wisely
> — better than you used to do.
> Pray and pray for courage
> Pray for sunshine, too,
> For somewhere in the great wide world
> A kidney waits for you.

Francie penned an asterisk at the last line and wrote in the margin: "Best bet: train crossings."

I think continually of those whom I've met or talked to in the course of this book. Leah and Michael appear to me in the living room that jiggles when the subway passes underneath. Jill's young face turns toward me, and I hope she's left her schizophrenic husband, finding the pain of leaving less than the pain of staying. Miriam fixes morning coffee for Daniel and watches the spring trees bud outside her window. Colman gives Krista her 6 A.M. wake-up call, and Kathy sits alone on the sands of her nearby beach while her children run into the water. Tom bakes cookies for his kids and tries not to notice small changes in Lisa. Alix and her youngest son, Dick, stamp their skis at the top of a snowy slope as she goes on trying to build the family that nature has railed so hard against. Laurie and Bill ride their Suzuki. Liz takes the heating pad off her knee and walks gingerly to the kitchen to put Carlo's potatoes in the oven. We are the solid, steady brother of a son not exactly prodigal but somewhat wasted. We may yet grow into the father, who opens his arms to both and feels joy.

They ran to the car with flowers and energy and excitement and, yes, happiness. Debbie drove the throughway halfway to Boston, and she and Kate talked and laughed all the way. One should always be outnumbered by teenagers. That way you don't give any boring lectures and you get to listen to them laugh instead. Outside Fenway Park, the Boston accents were as thick as the smell of hot and sweet sausages on the grill. Hawkers called, "Caps! Shirts! Get your Red Sox cap!" The metallic green lamps rose high over the wall of the stadium we were skirting on our way to Debbie's optometrist. Families emerged from the subway wearing Red Sox shirts; kids carried mitts and balls. Life moved and swelled around us and seemed good.

Ted's starting a short comic essay now. This weekend Seth telephoned to say he is studying Urdu. Perhaps his generation, with all its sense of doom, will move a little further toward saving the world. You don't build it in a day. I put *La Bohème* on the record player and went into the living room bay to water the paper whites that the kids gave Ted for his birthday. He sat at the dining room table reading the obituary column of the *Times* to find a name for a character in his essay.

"When I die," he called out, "don't have them send money to the Multiple Sclerosis Society. Tell them to send it to the Metropolitan Opera."

"When I die, they can mail mine to Fenway Park!" The paper whites were growing straight up out of their plastic pots, an inch tall.

*Appendix A*

# Useful Addresses and Telephone Numbers

## SOME NATIONAL ASSOCIATIONS, FOUNDATIONS, AND SOCIETIES

These societies are arranged alphabetically according to the capitalized key word. The national organizations for illnesses raise funds for research, provide information, and coordinate local chapters, which offer support groups. For groups not listed here, consult the *Encyclopedia of Associations* at your library.

Children of AGING Parents
2761 Trenton Road
Levittown, PA 19056
215-945-6900
This group also gives advice for adults with dependent spouses.

National Association of State Units on AGING
600 Maryland Avenue, SW, Suite 208
Washington, DC 20024
202-484-7182
If you're looking for an adult day care center and can't find one in your phone book's yellow pages, nor your area agency on aging in the front pages or blue pages, write or call for the address of your state unit on aging. Your state unit can direct you to an area agency and they will pinpoint local adult day care centers.

National Council on AGING
600 Maryland Avenue, SW, West Wing 100
Washington, DC 20024
202-479-1200

National ALZHEIMER'S DISEASE
  and Related Disorders Association
70 East Lake Street
Chicago, IL 60601
800-621-0379 or 312-853-3060

The ARTHRITIS Foundation
1314 Spring Street, NW
Atlanta, GA 30309
404-872-7100

American CANCER Society
4 West 35th Street
New York, NY 10001
212-736-3030

American DIABETES Association
1660 Duke Street
Alexandria, VA 22313
703-549-1500

The Concern for DYING
250 West 57th Street
New York, NY 10107
212-246-6962

National FUNERAL Directors Association
11121 West Oklahoma Avenue
Milwaukee, WI 53227
414-541-2500

GRAY PANTHERS
806 15th Street, NW, Suite 430
Washington, DC 20005
202-783-6226

American HEART Association
7320 Greenville Avenue
Dallas, TX 75231
214-750-5300

HEMLOCK Society
P.O. Box 66218
Los Angeles, CA 90066
213-391-1871
Derek Humphry's book *Let Me Die Before I Wake* was published by the society in 1982 and gives case histories of
self-deliveries, as well as a list of penal codes on assisted
suicide by state.

National HOSPICE Organization
1901 North Fort Myer Drive, Suite 902
Arlington, VA 22209
703-243-5900

IMPOTENCE Institute of America, Inc.
IMPOTENTS ANONYMOUS (I.A.)
I-ANON for Partners of Impotent Men
119 South Ruth Street
Maryville, TN 37801-5746
615-983-6064
This group will send not only a list of support groups in your
area but also a list of area urologists who deal with impotence.

National KIDNEY Foundation, Inc.
2 Park Avenue
New York, NY 10016
212-889-2210

National Senior Citizens LAW Center
2025 M Street, NW, Suite 400
Washington, DC 20036
202-887-5280

LEUKEMIA Society of America, Inc.
733 Third Avenue
New York, NY 10017
212-573-8484

American LUNG Association
1740 Broadway
New York, NY 10019
212-315-8700

The LUPUS Foundation of America, Inc.
1717 Massachusetts Avenue, NW, Suite 203
Washington, DC 20036
800-558-0121

The American LUPUS Society
23751 Madison Street
Torrance, CA 90505
213-373-1335

The National LUPUS ERYTHEMATOSUS Foundation
5430 Van Nuys Boulevard, Suite 206
Van Nuys, CA 91401
818-885-8787

National Alliance for the MENTALLY ILL
1901 North Fort Myer Avenue, Suite 500
Arlington, VA 22209
703-524-7600

The National MULTIPLE SCLEROSIS Society
205 East 42d Street
New York, NY 10017
212-986-3240

The MYASTHENIA GRAVIS Foundation
7–11 South Broadway
White Plains, NY 10601
914-328-1717

American PARKINSON'S DISEASE Association
116 John Street, Suite 417
New York, NY 10038
212-732-9550

PARKINSON'S DISEASE Foundation
Columbia Presbyterian Medical Center
650 West 168th Street
New York, NY 10032
212-923-4700

International POLIO Network
Gazette International Networking Institute
4502 Maryland Avenue
St. Louis, MO 63108
314-361-0475

STROKE Club International
805 12th Street
Galveston, TX 77550
403-762-1022

Older WOMEN'S LEAGUE (OWL)
1325 G Street, NW, Lower Level B
Washington, DC 20005
202-783-6686

FEDERAL AGENCIES

Office of Federal Contract Compliance Programs
US Department of Labor
200 Constitution Avenue, NW
Washington, DC 20210
202-523-9410

The United States Department of Health and Human Services
200 Independence Avenue, SW
Washington, DC 20201
202-245-6296

Public Health Service
200 Independence Avenue, SW
Washington, DC 20201
202-245-6867

*The National Institutes below foster and support ongoing research:*

National Institute of Mental Health
5600 Fishers Lane
Rockville, MD 20857
301-443-3606

National Institutes of Health
Bethesda, MD 20892
301-496-4000

National Cancer Institute
9000 Rockville Pike
Bethesda, MD 20892
800-4-CANCER or 301-496-5583

National Heart, Lung, and Blood Institute
7550 Wisconsin Avenue
Bethesda, MD 20892
301-496-4868

National Institute of Arthritis and Musculoskeletal and Skin Diseases
9000 Rockville Pike
Bethesda, MD 20892
301-496-3583

National Institute of Diabetes, Kidney and Digestive Disease
9000 Rockville Pike
Bethesda, MD 20892
301-496-3583

> National Digestive Diseases Education Information Clearing House
> 1255 23d Street, NW
> Washington, DC 20037
> 202-296-1138

> Kidney, Urologic, and Hematological Diseases
> 5333 Westbard Avenue
> Bethesda, MD 20892
> 301-496-7458

National Institute of Neurological and Communicative Disorders and Stroke
9000 Rockville Pike
Bethesda, MD 20892
301-496-5751

National Institute on Aging
9000 Rockville Pike
Bethesda, MD 20892
301-496-9265

INSURANCE COMPANIES OFFERING LONG-TERM CUSTODIAL COVERAGE

This list of companies offering nursing home coverage was provided by the Brookings Institution, 1775 Massachusetts Avenue, NW, Washington DC 20036, telephone 202-797-6266.

Call your own insurance agent to inquire or consult *Best's Agents Guide to Life Insurance Companies* at your library for addresses: Aetna, American Bankers, American Integrity, American International Group, American Republic, California Life, CNA, Colonial Penn, Columbia Life, Equitable Life, Fireman's Fund, Great Republic, Massachusetts Indemnity and Life Group Plan, Medico Life, National Foundation Equitable, Penn Treaty, Provider's Fidelity, Prudential, Sterling Life, Transport Life, United Equitable, World Life and Health.

Very recently, certain insurance companies have been experimenting with offering coverage for in-home custodial care. Among them are Metropolitan Life Insurance Company (which is trying a plan with an HMO in Seattle); Blue Cross of Washington and Alaska (trying another plan in Seattle); Blue Cross and Shield (trying plans in Kansas City, Missouri, and in Rochester, New York); the American Association of Retired Persons with the Prudential Insurance Company of America (trying an eight-state plan). Find out what new plans might be available to you.

Be sure to inquire about existing condition clauses and ultimate length of coverage.

MODEL PROGRAMS FOR CARE GIVERS OF THE SEVERELY DISABLED

Women Who Care
Box 692
Mill Valley, CA 94942
This group is writing *Women Take Care,* a collective account of the care giving they themselves have done.

The Family Survival Project
44 Page Street, Suite 600
San Francisco, CA 94102
415-626-6556
This group publishes a guide (1985) to more than one hundred care-giver support groups in California for Alzheimer's, stroke, multiple sclerosis, Parkinson's, Huntington's, and related disorders excluding head trauma.

The Natural Supports Program
Community Service Society of New York
105 East 22d Street
New York, NY 10010
212-254-8900

One of the nation's pioneer social service agencies, the Community Service Society focuses on aiding the poor and the disenfranchised; it offers some support groups for the families of the sick.

## National Well Spouses

We don't exist, but why not? If such a group would interest you, send a postcard (no letters!) to National Well Spouses, Box 100, Little, Brown and Company, 205 Lexington Avenue, New York, NY 10016. Give your name, address, telephone number, your spouse's illness and its severity (severe, moderate, mild), and both of your ages. If you live in a small town, give the nearest large city. You may or may not hear further, depending upon how many people respond with postcards.

*Appendix B*
# A Short, Sometimes Annotated, List of Books

Books referred to in more than one chapter appear under the first chapter in which they are mentioned.

CHAPTER 2: GETTING THE NEWS

John Rolland, "Toward a Psychosocial Typology of Chronic and Life-Threatening Illness," *Family Systems Medicine*, fall 1984. "Chronic Illness and the Life Cycle," in E. A. Carter and M. McGoldrick (Eds.), *The Family Life Cycle: A Framework for Family Therapy*, Gardner, 1987. "Chronic Illness and the Life Cycle: A Conceptual Framework," in *Family Process*, vol. 26, 1987.
Domeena Renshaw, "Sex and Depression: Coping with an Impotent Husband," *Sexual Medicine Today*, September 1981.

CHAPTER 4: THE ACUTE EMOTIONS

Mardi J. Horowitz, *Stress Response Syndromes*, Aronson, 2d ed., 1986.
Edward J. Speedling, *Heart Attack: The Family Response at Home and in the Hospital*, Tavistock, 1982. Top-notch objective look at what really happens when you get home.

CHAPTER 6: CHANGED DEPENDENCIES: MAMA (OR PAPA) AND BABY

Myron Eisenberg, LaFaye C. Sutkin, and Mary A. Jansen (Eds.), *Chronic Illness and Disability through the Life Span,* Springer, 1984.

Michael Elkin, *Families under the Influence,* Norton, 1984.

H. A. Lange and T. Jackubowsky, *Responsible Assertive Behavior: Cognitive–Behavioral Procedures for Trainers,* University of Illinois Press, 1976. If you want to read about assertion, this is the basic book.

Harriet Goldhor Lerner, *The Dance of Anger: A Woman's Guide to Changing the Patterns of Intimate Relationships,* Harper and Row, 1985. Dr. Lerner tells how to get out of the underfunctioning and overfunctioning circle.

Katherine Newman, *Falling from Grace: The Meaning of Downward Mobility in American Culture,* Free Press, to be published in 1988.

Sharon Wegscheider, *Another Chance,* Science and Behavior, 1981.

CHAPTER 8: THE CHRONIC EMOTIONS

Carroll E. Izard, Jerome Kagan, and Robert B. Zajonc (Eds.), *Emotion, Cognition, and Behavior,* Cambridge University Press, 1984. The remarks on the evolutionary function of emotions come from Dr. Kagan's chapter "The Idea of Emotion in Human Development."

Martha Weinman Lear, *Heartsounds,* Simon and Schuster, 1980. Does this compelling account describe a "long acute" or a "short chronic" illness? Read and decide.

Robert and Suzanne Massie, *Journey,* Knopf, 1973.

CHAPTER 10: FIGHTING OFF THE GURUS

Walter Cannon, *Bodily Changes in Pain, Hunger, Fear and Rage,* 2d ed., Charles Branford, 1953.

Barrie R. Cassileth, Edward J. Lusk, David S. Miller, Lorraine L. Brown, and Clifford Miller, "Psychosocial Correlates of Survival in Advanced Malignant Disease?," *The New England Journal of Medicine,* no. 312: June 13, 1985.

O. Carl Simonton and Stephanie Matthews-Simonton,

*Getting Well Again*, J. P. Tarcher, 1978, distributed by St. Martin's Press.

CHAPTER 14: ACTS OF RESCUE (AND WHAT ABOUT THAT AFFAIR?)

Meyer Friedman, M.D., and Ray H. Rosenman, M.D., *Type A Behavior and Your Heart*, Knopf, 1974.

Clara Livsey, "Physical Illness and Family Dynamics," in Paul W. Power and Arthur E. Dell Orto (Eds.), *Role of the Family in the Rehabilitation of the Physically Disabled*, University Park Press, 1980.

Quentin Regestein, with James R. Rechs, *Sound Sleep*, Simon and Schuster, 1980. This is a good guide to dealing with insomnia.

*University of California, Berkeley, Wellness Letter*, vol. 2, issue 5, February 1986.

CHAPTER 16: HOW DEVASTATING ILLNESS DEVASTATES A FAMILY

Heidi I. Hartmann, "The Family as the Locus of Gender, Class, and Political Struggle: The Example of Housework," *Signs*, vol. 6, no. 3, 1981.

David Rintell, "Children of Chronically Ill Parents: Family Context and Child Adjustment," Ed.D. Thesis, Boston University, University Microfilm, 1985.

CHAPTER 18: EVERYDAY MARRIAGE, EVERYDAY AGING

Florence Kaslow, "Portrait of a Healthy Couple," *Psychiatric Clinics*, vol. 5, no. 3, December 1982.

J. M. Lewis, W. R. Beavers, J. T. Gosset, and V. A. Phillips, *No Single Thread: Psychological Health in Family Systems*, Brunner/Mazel, 1976.

Susan Rako and Harvey Mazer (Eds.), *Semrad: The Heart of a Therapist*, Jason Aronson, 1980.

CHAPTER 20: TILL DEATH DOES OR DOESN'T US PART

Richard S. Blacher, "Reaction to Chronic Illness," in Bernard Schoenberg, Arthur C. Carr, David Peretz, and Austin H.

Kutscher (Eds.), *Loss and Grief: Psychological Management*, Columbia University Press, 1970.

Vanda Colman, with the assistance of Tish Sommers and Fran Leonard, "Gray Paper No. 7, Issues for Action: "Till Death Do Us Part: Caregiving Wives of Severely Disabled Husbands," Older Women's League, Washington, 1982.

Margaret Gold, *Life Support: Families Speak About Hospital, Hospice and Home Care for the Fatally Ill*, Institute of Consumer Policy Research, Consumers Union Fd., 1983. For a four-dollar condensation, contact the Institute at 256 Washington Street, Mount Vernon, New York, NY 10553.

Derek Humphry, *Jean's Way*, Quartet Books, 1978, and *Let Me Die Before I Wake: Hemlock's Book of Self-Deliverance for the Dying*, The Hemlock Society, 1981 and 1982.

Lois Barclay Murphy, *The Home Hospital, How a Family Can Cope with Catastrophic Illness*, Basic Books, 1982. If you want and can afford to nurse at home.

Robyn Stone, Gail Lee Cafferata, and Judith Sangl, "Caregivers of the Frail Elderly: A National Profile," US Department of Health and Human Services. This report examines data from the 1982 National Long-term Care Survey and reports that most of the care givers of the disabled elderly are women; 13 percent are husbands.

David Young, *Earthshine*, Wesleyan University Press, to be published in 1988. In this collection will appear "Nine Deaths," David Young's poem for his wife, Chloe.

# Index

abstention from sex, 237–238
acute emotions, 47–54, 76–77, 217
acute illness, 21
adult day care, 79, 285
aging, 234
  chronic illness and, 228, 246
  sex and, 106
  and well spouse, 190
Aging, National Association of State
    Units on, 301
Aging, National Council on, 302
Aging, National Institute on, 306
Aging Parents, Children of, 301
AIDS, 30
alcohol, 188–189
Alcoholics Anonymous, 163
alcoholism, 81–83
alienation, children's feelings of,
  248
ALS. *See* amylateral sclerosis
Alzheimer's disease, 22, 25,
    170–171, 259, 265–268, 269,
    270–271, 280–281, 290, 297
  family support groups, 170–172
  Family Survival Project, 171–172,
    307
  loss of autonomy, 238
  sexual desires of patients, 105,
    106
Alzheimer's Disease and Related
    Disorders Association,
    National, 302
ambivalence, 30, 101

  of children, 213–214
  of well spouse, 30, 101, 109, 189
American Psychiatric Association,
  160
Amigo (wheelchair), 201–203, 205
amylateral sclerosis, 24, 77, 118
anger, 238
  children's feelings of, 129,
    173–174, 211–212, 213, 215, 221,
    248
  guilt and, 115
  ill spouse's feelings of, 113–115,
    209
  of married couples, 237, 244
  well spouse's feelings of, 50, 65,
    66, 68–69, 86, 88, 113–115, 136,
    150, 161, 170, 182, 183, 209,
    250–252, 276–277
annoyance, well spouse's feelings
  of, 102, 112–113, 181
anxiety, 147
  of children, 215
  and family, 216
  relaxation techniques for, 160–161
  and well spouse, 117, 118–119,
    182
arthritis, 114, 139–141
  as result of stress, 135
Arthritis and Musculoskeletal and
    Skin Diseases, National Insti-
    tute of, 306
Arthritis Foundation, 166–167, 302
assertion, 86

I.A. *See* Impotents Anonymous
I-ANON, 26, 303
ill spouse
  aging and, 228
  ambivalence of, 30
  anger and, 113–115, 209
  blame and, 32–34
  checklist for, 244–245
  communication and, 86, 244–245
  complaining by, 182
  consideration of well spouse,
    244–245
  courage of, 212
  death of, 288
  denial by, 32–34, 81, 97–98, 198,
    272
  dependencies of, 112, 212,
    224–225, 244, 246
  depression and, 98, 209, 219–222,
    241
  desire for independence of, 241
  effects of automatic aid on, 85–86
  emotions of, 244–245
  endurance of, 212
  fears of, 30, 66, 210, 244
  friends and, 92–93
  guilt feelings of, 244
  incapacitation and, 30
  infantile behavior of, 83–84, 137,
    244
  isolation, feelings of, 30, 32–34,
    113, 115–116, 273
  jealousy of, 113
  job, loss of, and, 44–46, 53, 54,
    55–56, 76, 78–79
  needs of, 68, 269–271
  reactions upon initial diagnosis,
    24–34
  response to problems of well
    spouse, 86
  self-orientation and, 80
  stress and, 57–58
  support groups for, 163–171
IMA. *See* individual medical
    accounts
impotence, 4–10, 15–16, 26–27, 33
  diabetes and, 164
  implants, 168–170
  injection program, 168–170
  mental illness and, 219
  multiple sclerosis and, 39–40
  well spouse and, 194
  wife's reaction to, 27, 106,
    169–170

Impotence Institute of America,
    Inc., 26, 303
Impotents Anonymous (I.A.), 26,
    168–169, 303
Imuran, 132, 133, 147
incapacitation, 30
incompetency, 170, 287
independence, 224
  children's need for, 213, 235
  ill spouse's desire for, 241
  in marriage, 236
individual medical accounts, 268
individual therapy
  long-term, 160–161
  short-term, 161
inequality, feelings of, 107
infantile behavior, 57, 84–85, 137,
    245
information workshops, 163–166
insomnia, 189, 190
insurance, 79, 266–267. *See also*
    Medicaid; Medicare
  companies, 306–307
  custodial care, 268, 287–288
  disability, 18, 62
  federal disability, 99–100
  group health, 54
  individual health, 54
  life, 266, 286–287
  Medicare, 52
  nursing homes and, 285
  private, 98–100, 131, 264
  therapy and, 161
intensive care units, 50–51
isolation, 32–34, 52
  children's feelings of, 223
  ill spouse's feelings of, 30, 32–34,
    113, 115–116, 273
  well spouse's feelings of, 26,
    32–34, 43–44, 113, 115–116, 169,
    194, 259

jealousy, 87
  children's feelings of, 213
  ill spouse's feelings of, 113
  well spouse's feelings of, 87, 102,
    111–112, 113
*Jean's Way* (Humphry), 255
job
  ill spouse's loss of, 44–46, 53, 54,
    55–56, 76, 78–79
  well spouse's, 44–46, 65, 76–77
*Journey* (Massie), 119
Jungian therapists, 162

powerlessness, of the well spouse, 137
privacy, in marriage, 237
psychiatric social workers, 162
psychiatry, 159–160, 162
psychoanalysis, 160–161
psychotherapy, 138–139, 146–147, 150, 157–158, 209
Public Health Service, 305

record keeping, 79
Regestein, Quentin, 189
Rehabilitation Act (1973), 53
rejection, well spouse's fear of, 194
relaxation techniques, 160–161, 187
religion, 192–193, 232, 251, 269
  children and, 214
relocating, 57–74, 249
remission, 69, 139, 141
Renshaw, Domeena, 27, 106
resentment
  therapy and, 161
  well spouse's feelings of, 107, 140
resignation, well spouse's feelings of, 148
respite care, 260, 285–286
responsibility, well spouse's feelings of, 48, 162
resuscitation, 278–279, 281, 288
Retired Persons, American Association of, 263
retirement, 82–83
  forced, 53
rheumatoid arthritis, 22, 137
Rintell, David, 215–216
role reversal, 237. See also sex roles
Rolland, John, 27–29, 104

sacrifice, 101
sadness, 117
  children's feelings of, 129
  at loss of companion, xi
  well spouse's feelings of, 102–107, 261, 276, 297–298
Sammons, James H., 278
Satir, Virginia, 81
schizophrenia, 25. See also mental illness
Seconal, 279
self-denial, 252
self-esteem, 117, 137
self-pity, 146
Semrad, Elvin, 236

sense of self, well spouse's loss of, 55–76, 80–88, 102, 175, 180, 254
separation
  children's need for, 214
  emotional, 228
sex
  and aging, 106
  health professionals' methods of dealing with, 106
  extramarital, 194–196, 229, 237–238
  therapy, 10, 26, 161
sex roles, 56–57, 60, 83–84, 215, 237
sexual dysfunction, 26, 161
sexual identity, 103–107
sexual relationship, 102–107, 194–196, 235–236, 237
shame, children's feelings of, 213
shock, 29
shunts, 29
Simonton, O. Carl, 135–136
situational pain, 162
sleep, well spouse's need for, 117, 189
sleeping arrangements, changing, 189
smoking, 242–243
social life, decrease in, 111, 115–116, 175
Social Security, 54, 131, 132, 266, 267, 283, 287. See also Medicaid; Medicare; Supplemental Security Income
societies for chronic illnesses, 301–305
"soft death," 280
sorrow, 119, 170, 238. See also sadness
Specific Personality Theory, 135
speech problems, 15
speech therapy, 269, 283
Speedling, Edward J., 50–52, 83
spending down, 285. See also financial hardships; spousal impoverishment
spinal cord injury, course of, 29–30
spinal tap, 15, 18
spousal impoverishment, 265–268, 287. See also financial hardships; spending down
spouse. See ill spouse; well spouse
Stark, Fortney, 264
stress, 135–142. See also tension
  and bereavement, 136

stress (*continued*)
    children's feelings of, 175
    and the ill spouse, 57–58
    illnesses related to, 189–190
    polarized emotions and, 84–85
    reactions to, 84–85
    and the well spouse, 136–137
stress response, 135
stroke, 22, 23, 108, 192, 204–205,
        259, 266, 269, 307
    course of, 29–30
    and loss of autonomy, 238
Stroke Club International, 305
suicide, 253, 254–257, 279–281, 288,
        303
    assisted, 279–281
    well spouse's thoughts of, 118
Supplemental Security Income, 282,
        283, 284. *See also* Social Security
support groups, 159, 163–172,
        250–252, 258–262, 282. *See also*
        therapy
    family, 170–172
sympathetic response, 135

tension, 141, 248–249. *See also* stress
therapy, 159–172. *See also* support
        groups
    behavioral, 160–161
    cognitive, 160
    couples, 161, 162
    family, 28, 127–130, 161–162,
        223
    group, 9, 11, 39, 162
    individual, 160–161
    marital, 105
    in nursing homes, 269–271
    occupational, 269
    physical, 269, 283
    psychotherapy, 146–147, 150,
        157–158
    selecting, 159–160
    sex, 10, 26, 161
    speech, 269, 283
Thoreson, Carl, 188
thyroiditis, 137
*Till Death Do Us Part: Caregiving
    Wives of Severely Disabled Hus-
    bands* (Colman), 258
time, perceptions of, 27–28, 41, 114
trust, assault to, 48, 244

ulcerative colitis, course of, 29–30
ulcers, 29

unemployment, 44–46, 53, 54,
        55–56, 76, 78–79, 91, 93

vacations, 202
values, of the married couple, 237,
        239
Veterans Administration, 282
vision problems, 15. *See also* blind-
        ness
visiting nurse, 263, 286

Waxman, Henry A., 265
Weakest Link Theory, 135
Wegscheider, Sharon, 81
well spouse
    adjustments and, 101
    aging and, 190, 228
    ambivalence and, 30, 101, 109,
        189
    anger and, 50, 65, 66, 68–69,
        86, 88, 113–115, 136, 150, 161,
        170, 182, 183, 209, 250–252,
        276–277
    annoyance and, 102, 112–113, 181
    anticipatory grief and, 30, 225,
        271, 274
    anxiety and, 117, 118–119, 147,
        182
    assertion of, 86
    automatic aid and, 85–86
    and autonomy of ill spouse,
        83–86
    betrayal, feelings of, 73
    blame and, 32–34, 137–138
    boredom with disease and, 113,
        116, 161, 261
    career of, 44–46, 65, 76–77,
        144–145, 197
    checklist for, 245–246
    consideration of ill spouse,
        245–246
    death of, 287
    defensiveness toward ill spouse,
        69
    deferring gratification, 82
    denial and, 32–34, 59–60, 97, 259
    depression and, 50, 117–118, 147,
        148, 187, 209
    deprivation of pleasure, 88
    diagnosis, reactions to, 24–34
    disappointment, feelings of, 140,
        170, 181
    emotional contact and, 85
    empathy and, 239–244, 245